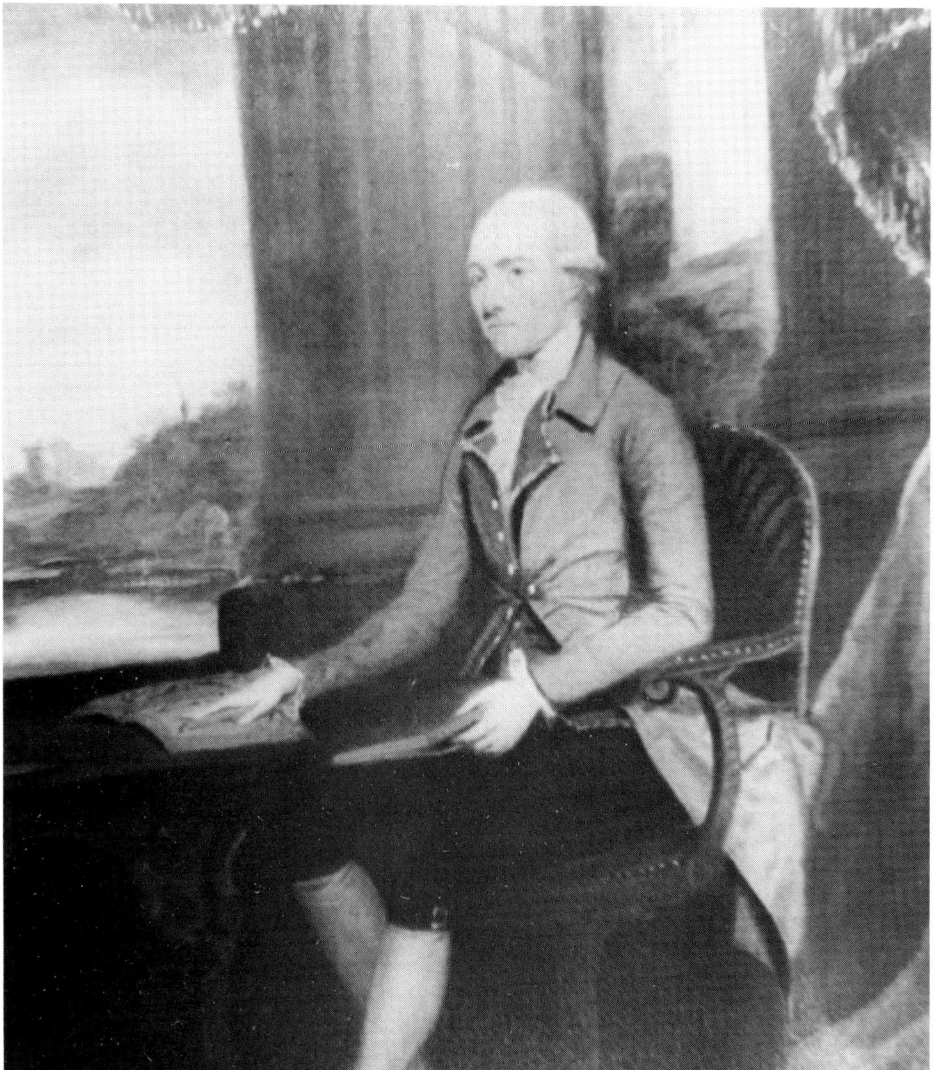

Plate 1: William Brownrigg. Artist unknown.
(Reproduced with permission of the West Cumberland Hospital, Whitehaven.)

THE MEDICAL CASEBOOK OF WILLIAM BROWNRIGG, M.D., F.R.S. (1712–1800) OF THE TOWN OF WHITEHAVEN IN CUMBERLAND

(*Medical History*, Supplement No. 13)

THE MEDICAL CASEBOOK OF WILLIAM BROWNRIGG, M.D., F.R.S. (1712–1800) OF THE TOWN OF WHITEHAVEN IN CUMBERLAND

edited and translated by

JEAN E. WARD and JOAN YELL

(*Medical History*, Supplement No. 13)

LONDON
WELLCOME INSTITUTE FOR THE HISTORY OF MEDICINE
1993

ISBN 0 85484 125 3

Supplements to *Medical History* may be obtained by post from Professional and Scientific Publications, BMA House, Tavistock Square, London WC1H 9JR.

CONTENTS

ACKNOWLEDGEMENTS

We would like to thank Mr A. Welton and Mr S. White of Carlisle Library for permission to publish the Casebook; Mr H. Fancy of Whitehaven Museum and Miss A. Dick of Whitehaven Library for local matters; Mr D. Bowcock of Cumbria County Record Office, Carlisle; Miss M. E. Burkett of Isel Hall; Mr H. Brownrigg of London; the Librarian of the Royal College of Physicians of Edinburgh; Mr G. Gunthorpe of the British Society for the History of Pharmacy; Prof. J. V. Beckett of Nottingham; Dr David Harley of Oxford; Prof. V. Nutton, Prof. Roy Porter, and Dr C. Stevenson of the Wellcome Institute; Mrs J. Arnott and Mrs K. Muldoon for typing the manuscript.

EDITORS' NOTE

The Casebook has been transcribed as it lies, with the spelling and punctuation of the English sections preserved. Numbers have been allocated to the cases by the editors to aid reference. The prescriptions have been indented and inserted in the text at the correct locations. Editorial interpolations are inserted between square brackets or provided in footnotes.

INTRODUCTION

William Brownrigg (1712–1800) was an accomplished physician, scientist and polymath who spent his life in medical practice in the town of Whitehaven in the County of Cumberland. An excellent biography of the man has been produced by J. V. Beckett,[1] but his medical career has been largely neglected. It is obvious that, had he moved to London instead of remaining in such a remote area, his experiments would have ensured him a place as one of the greatest intellects of the eighteenth century.

BIOGRAPHY

He was born on March 13th, 1712 at High Close Hall, Plumbland, near Aspatria, the eldest son of George Brownrigg, a small country landowner who had married his cousin Mary. The family eventually grew to three boys and four girls, and William as the eldest received a good education, firstly at the church schools of Crosthwaite, Keswick and Isel, Cockermouth. By the age of thirteen, he showed such promise as a scholar that his family paid for private tuition in Greek and Latin from the Vicar of Bridekirk.[2] At fifteen, he was apprenticed to a surgeon/apothecary of Carlisle, John Atkinson, for a period of five years at £40 per annum,[3] but Brownrigg continued to expand his education with tuition in Greek, Latin, French, Euclid, arithmetic and mathematics. On the completion of his apprenticeship and supported by his family and an inheritance of property from his grandfather, he then went to London and resided two years with a surgeon, Mr. Barnwilt, to increase his knowledge of pharmacy and the London method of curing disease.

In 1733, there was no academic institution in Britain where medicine was regarded as an important study, and Brownrigg, like many other British students, was forced to go abroad to study under the leading teachers of the era. Some of these were to be found in Leiden, drawn by the reputation of the aged, but still illustrious Hermann Boerhaave (1668–1738), Professor of Botany and Clinical Medicine. In the small Caecilia Hospital, he taught the value of clinical observation to students for over twenty years, and, by the time William Brownrigg reached Leiden as one of 25 matriculations,[4] graduates included Albrecht von Haller of the University of Göttingen, Linnaeus of Uppsala, Monro Primus of Edinburgh and Gerhard van Swieten, later founder of the Old Vienna School of Medicine.[5] In the three years of residency at Leiden, Brownrigg studied Physick with Boerhaave, Anatomy with Albinus, Botany with Van Royen and Experimental Philosophy with 'sGravesande, and in 1736 was awarded his doctorate on the presentation of a thesis 'De praxi medici ineunda'.[6] This was a set of precepts which physicians should employ in the treatment of their patients, including ". . . heads of discussion with regards to the state of the air, that of the climate and

[1] J. V. Beckett, 'Dr William Brownrigg FRS. Physician, chemist and country gentleman', *Notes and Records of the Royal Society of London*, 1976–7, **21**: 255–71.

[2] Manuscript sheet in Brownrigg's own hand entitled, 'W. Brownrigg, some occurrencies of his life and dates of ye same', Carlisle Record Office (hereafter CRO), DX/448/53.

[3] P. J. Wallis and R. V. Wallis, *Eighteenth century medics: subscriptions, licenses, apprenticeships*, Newcastle upon Tyne, Project for Historical Biobibliography, 1985.

[4] E. Ashworth Underwood, *Boerhaave's men at Leyden and after*, Edinburgh University Press, 1977, p. 20.

[5] Van Swieten (1700–1772) began his work in Vienna in 1745.

[6] J. E. Kroon, 'Boerhaave as professor-promoter', *Janus*, 1918, **23**: 291–311.

other contingencies affecting the place where the physician proposes to reside. To these are appended useful rules and judicious advice for the assistance and direction of medical students, relative to the characteristic temperament and constitution of its inhabitants; their mode of living; their particular articles of diet; the diseases and infirmities to which they are liable; and the means, which have been proved from experience, to be able to be adequate to their immediate relief or permanent removal."[7]

In January 1737, he sailed from Hellevoitsluis to Harwich and then travelled to Whitehaven to join Richard Senhouse, an apothecary and a Leiden graduate. When Senhouse died in October of that year,[8] the 25-year-old doctor continued alone with his patron's patients and remained in Whitehaven as a physician until the late 1760s. There were other doctors of various sorts in the town during this period (Appendix I) and many augmented their incomes by instructing apprentices. Senhouse had two,[9] but Brownrigg occupied himself with his scientific work and had no occasion to instruct others. He rented a modest house at 24 Queen Street[10] with three stories, a cellar and attic, the ground floor of which would have had his public consulting room. In 1741, he married Mary, the daughter of John Spedding, Sir James Lowther's estate agent,[11] and through her, began a close association in scientific work with her uncle, Carlisle, who was colliery steward. Brownrigg and Carlisle Spedding began to experiment on the dangerous fire and choke damps which bedevilled all the coal workings in Whitehaven and caused regular loss of life, such as the explosion at Corporal Pit in 1737 which killed 21 men, 1 woman and 3 horses. Light underground was normally supplied by tallow candles which gave no warning of the presence of lethal gases. The explosive nature of the air was demonstrated to the Royal Society by Sir James Lowther in 1741, using bladders filled with the mixture by Spedding and Brownrigg. They devised a safer method of lighting the dangerous pits with the invention of the Steel Mill: this had two rotating wheels, against one of which was held a flint to produce a shower of sparks. These were thought (wrongly) to be less liable to ignite the fire damp, but did give some warning of the presence of gases by a change of colour, and the device was widely adopted in mines until the invention of the Davy Safety Lamp.

In 1742, Sir James Lowther nominated William Brownrigg as a Fellow of the Royal Society in recognition of his work on the fire damp, paying the twenty-two guineas for his life membership.[12] In 1743 Spedding and Brownrigg persuaded Sir James Lowther to finance the construction of a small shed, and they rented the damp air from nearby Pedlar Pit, which was piped into this laboratory.[13] Here Brownrigg discovered the relationship between barometric pressure and the quantity of fire damp, allowing him to advise

[7] J. Dixon, *The literary life of William Brownrigg MD, FRS*, London, Longman & Rees, 1801, p. 3.
[8] Will of Richard Senhouse, Lancashire Record Office, WRW.C.
[9] Leopold Smith and William Laithes, as recorded in Wallis and Wallis, *Eighteenth century medics.*
[10] Recorded in the Whitehaven census of 1762. The house was owned by Mrs. Peggy Spedding and the plan is described in *Whitehaven 1660–1800*, by Sylvia Collier and Sarah Pearson, Royal Commission on Historical Monuments, London, HMSO, 1991, p. 126.
[11] Marriage settlement of William and Mary Brownrigg 1741, CRO, DX/448/12. They never had any children, and Mary lived until 1794. A contemporary described her as "an agreeable, clever woman but very vain and extravagant".
[12] Lowther to Spedding, letters, 20 and 29 May 1742, CRO, D/Lons/W. Sir James Lowther lived up to his reputation for meanness, however, as he recouped the membership fee from Brownrigg through John Spedding later in 1742.
[13] Estate Memoranda Books 1743, CRO, D/Lons/W.

Spedding on the safest periods for underground work in the pits.[14] The doctor also treated victims of these explosions, for in a letter to his friend Sir John Pringle, he stated: "Those who are burnt by fire damp in the coal pits in Cumberland are successfully treated with constant unctions of salad oil for the first 24 hours; that is, as soon as the skin dries some more oil is rubbed upon all the burn parts; afterwards the sores are dressed with cereates, softened with oil . . . the patients always complained of being cold during the first day or so, directed the oil to be warmed".[15] Pringle also noted Brownrigg's observation on a collier's health, which seemed curious from one who was such an acute observer of physical condition: ". . . in Cumberland, and he believed in other parts, the Coaliers are in general among the healthiest of the common people, unless when unguardedly exposing themselves to the cold air, after coming sweating from their work they are seized with some inflammatory disease. But that they suffered nothing from the air of the pits, except when either a fire damp or choak damp prevailed. That he [Brownrigg] once knew a weakly shoemaker, pale and asthmatic, become strong and healthful, by changing his trade for that of a coalier . . .".[16]

Apart from his medical and scientific work, Brownrigg involved himself in several local business enterprises. He invested in a local iron ore venture with leading merchants of Whitehaven, leased Skiddaw Forest from the Duke of Somerset with a view to exploiting the timber, and inherited a share in the Whitehaven Ropery on the death of his father-in-law, John Spedding. His connection with the Lowther family led him to act as agent for Sir James in political matters and to obtain the sinecure posts of Patent Searcher at Port Carlisle and Receiver General of Government Taxes for Cumberland and Westmorland. Some of his income from these was invested in the Keswick Turnpike Trust and the purchase of land at Ormathwaite near Keswick. His scientific work continued in tandem with his medical practice. In 1748, he wrote a book on *The art of making common salt*,[17] and was given a sample of the "Platina di Pinto" or Platinum by his brother-in-law, Charles Wood,[18] on which he experimented before presenting it to the Royal Society in 1741. After inheriting his father's estate at Millbeck and Ormathwaite, Keswick, in 1760, he still retained an interest in Whitehaven's health, but his new wealth allowed him to travel to Spa in Belgium in 1765 to carry out experiments on its mineral waters. He concluded, in a paper to the Royal Society,[19] that the evolution of "fixed air" from Spa water began at 110°F and that the "air" kept the earthy and metallic ingredients of the water in solution. In recognition of this, and also of his past work, the Royal Society awarded him the Copley Gold Medal in 1766 for his outstanding contribution to science.

He spent more time in semi-retirement at Ormathwaite from 1770 onwards, improving and enlarging the house and building an elaborate laboratory where he continued with his

[14] Lowther to Spedding, letters, 20 December 1744, CRO, D/Lons/W.

[15] Sir John Pringle, *Annotations MS*, vol. 1, 313, Royal College of Physicians, Edinburgh.

[16] Ibid., vol. 9, p. 380.

[17] This was written when salt imports were threatened by war, and he advocated how it might be done cheaply on a local basis, employing former sailors. This encouraged Sir James Lowther to build saltpans next to Saltom Pit. An abridgement was made of this book by the Royal Society and read there in June 1748. It was regarded as the most important technical paper read there in fifty years.

[18] Charles Wood married Brownrigg's widowed sister who had returned from Jamaica also. The sample came from Cartagena and was the first known arrival of that metal in England.

[19] 'Enquiries into the mineral elastic spirit or air contained in the Spa water; as well as into the mephitic qualities of this spirit', *Phil. Trans. R. Soc.*, 1765, **55**: 218–35.

experiments. He maintained an interest in geology, wrote a history of Cumberland, and encouraged the early tourists to visit the area.[20] He continued to correspond with medical men in other areas of Britain, and when plague appeared to be threatening the country in 1771, he wrote a paper on his own experiences of "Gaol Fever".[21] He was visited at Ormathwaite by Sir John Pringle and Benjamin Franklin in 1772, who were conducted down the Whitehaven mines by James Spedding, the son of Brownrigg's old colleague, Carlisle. Later they experimented with the effect of oil on the turbulent waves of Derwentwater.[22]

Having spent a great deal of money on estate improvements and building up a fine art collection in his later years,[23] Brownrigg accumulated debts of over £8,000 by 1787. A mortgage on the estate and the remaining money were paid by his nephew Anthony Benn, on condition that, when Brownrigg and his wife died, Benn should inherit the estate. The 1790s saw the death of the doctor's wife, which accelerated a rapid mental decline. His own funeral in 1800 was attended by many local dignitaries and three local baronets were pall-bearers. Mr Dixon, his successor in Whitehaven, not only wrote *The Literary Life of William Brownrigg* but also contributed a fulsome obituary in the *Gentleman's Magazine* to this "monument of departed genius".[24]

THE MANUSCRIPT

The Casebook of Dr. Brownrigg is in the Jacksonian Collection of Carlisle Library, Cumbria.[25] It measures 33 cm × 21 cm and is bound in brown marbled board with a leather spine, and, although in reasonable condition, about 40 pages have been carefully cut out towards the back of the volume. The book contains a variety of cases, observations and letters dating from 1737 to 1742. The case histories are arranged on one side of a divided page, and are balanced by the prescriptions on the other (Plate 3), with all cases written in Latin. English is used for some observations (e.g. on Mrs Stephens' Medicine) and also in a number of copy letters to and from other British physicians. Several small loose sheets are interspersed throughout the volume, a few of which have been firmly attached by sealing wax, as was also a page from the *Newcastle Courant* (see Plate 4). Most of the entries were written by Brownrigg, but two other hands can be discerned and a comparison with other documents suggests that Brownrigg's wife may have written some of the copy correspondence, e.g. the letters from Gilchrest, Hay, Monro and Carlyle.[26] Only one

[20] He encouraged the author of the first major tourist volume relating to the Lake District, Father Thomas West, who was given many ideas for his *Guide to the lakes* (published in 1778) when he visited Brownrigg at Ormathwaite.

[21] *Considerations on the means of preventing the communication of pestilential contagion and the eradicating of it in infected places*, London, Lockyer Davis, 1771.

[22] 'On the stilling of waves by means of oil', *Phil. Trans. R. Soc.*, 1774, **64**: 445–60. Franklin continued to correspond with Brownrigg and personal letters are still extant in private hands.

[23] *Catalogue of the Ormathwaite sale*, 1804. In the collection of pictures were two Rembrandts, two Raphaels, a Rubens and a Poussin. The entire art collection was probably worth in excess of £100,000 in eighteenth-century money.

[24] *Gentleman's Magazine*, 1800, pp. 386–8.

[25] MS. E104, Jacksonian Collection, Carlisle Library. We are indebted to the Library for permission to publish the Casebook, and particularly to Mr Stephen White, the Local History Librarian. We also acknowledge the assistance of Mr Harry Fancy of Whitehaven Museum in making the document available for study in secure conditions.

[26] CRO, letter from Mary Brownrigg, 1780.

original letter, that of Dr. Simpson, has been included, and that only because Brownrigg drafted his reply on the back of it. Entries are made in fairly strict chronological order, but it is obvious that this Casebook is only an abstract from his daily records of some of his most interesting cases, and these tend to be grouped together according to the particular conditions. Perhaps this volume was prepared as a basis for a textbook which was never published, as it includes at least one lengthy dissertation, on haemorrhoids, of Brownrigg's own composition, based on practical experience and written references which he had carefully assembled.

THE TOWN AND BROWNRIGG'S PATIENTS

By 1737, the year of Brownrigg's arrival in Whitehaven, the town was one of the most prosperous ports in Britain. The Lowther family had owned the town area and the surrounding Manor of St Bees since 1630, and as largely absentee landlords had received income from farms and mineral holdings. At the end of the seventeenth century, the coal measures were little exploited, but when Sir James Lowther inherited the estate in 1706, there followed such an expansion that, by the 1750s, Whitehaven produced and exported over 80 per cent of all the coal for Dublin.[27] James Lowther spent most of his time in London but kept in touch with events in the port through a detailed correspondence with his local agents. Regarded as a miserly bachelor by his peers,[28] Lowther never failed to invest capital in his coal enterprises and the expansion of the harbour to ease the coal trade.

The most remarkable of his local advisers were the Spedding brothers, sons of one of the poorer tenant farmers on the estate. John Spedding was probably educated at a school founded by Sir John to teach navigation and mathematics to boys who wanted to enter the sea trade. He became a servant at the Flatt,[29] and when Sir James inherited from his father, Sir John, Spedding was enlisted as his spy to report on the activities of John Gale the colliery agent. Detailed letters and accounts passed between master and servant, often several times a week and in a shorthand code, informing Sir James of all Gale's activities. These gradually damned the colliery agent by referring to cash not accounted for in the coal loadings at the harbour and debts mounting in Gale's name, until in 1707, he was dismissed on suspicion of embezzlement and his position passed to the devious John Spedding.[30] Spedding purchased more coal-bearing land on behalf of his master and thwarted other local landowners' attempts to encroach on the Lowther monopoly by sabotaging workings and enticing colliers away with higher wages. He promoted Sir James's interest so well that in 1730 he became estate agent and care of the collieries was passed to his brother Carlisle, a gifted engineer who sank many deep pits and pioneered in the mines the use of modern equipment such as the "Scotch" Gin and the Newcomen Steam Engine.

Both Sir John and Sir James wished to see the town prosper, and detailed plans were drawn up for a steady expansion along a grid network of streets. Plots were leased or sold at a low rate to the merchants and ships' captains, and houses with fine interior fittings and

[27] J. V. Beckett, *Coal and tobacco*, Cambridge University Press, 1981.

[28] Ibid., pp. 17, 19.

[29] A mansion built by Sir George Fletcher of Hutton, and acquired by Sir John in 1675, then subsequently enlarged.

[30] The unsavoury spying procedure is set down in a series of letters, partly in cipher, in the Carlisle Record Office (D/Lons). John Spedding was, in fact, Gale's nephew.

spacious gardens were soon to be seen between the Flatt and the harbour.[31] The merchants accumulated wealth through the expanding port, not from the poor agricultural hinterland of the town. Trade went on between Whitehaven and Europe, but the most prosperous commerce was in coal to Ireland. The Lowthers never owned the coal ships but allowed the merchants to risk the shipbuilding finance, and then sold them the coal at a dictated rate. Many merchants wholly or partly owned ships which also traded across the Atlantic to the West Indies and the American colonies. By 1737 tobacco, spirits, sugar and spices were all being stored in the large warehouses built next to the merchants' houses. Many owned land in the colonies and some even participated in the lucrative but uncertain slave trade.[32] Such men built and lived in the town depicted in 1738 by Matthias Rhead in a painting *A bird's eye view of Whitehaven*. This shows the layout of wide streets, elegant houses and two fine churches.[33] Industry grew in the town based on trade imports, the coal mines and the harbour, and in the early years of Brownrigg's Casebook there were already a ropeworks, shipbuilding, a glassworks, brewery and sugarhouse. As people were drawn to the flourishing town, the spacious nature of the plan was altered, with plots being sub-divided, and gardens built over by newer dwellings. People were often housed in attics and cellars of large houses, rented out by their owners.[34]

The Town Book, a record of the Manorial Court of St Bees from 1702–1782,[35] recorded many infringements of town laws which were detrimental to general public health. Pavements were often in bad repair, cellars were dug without regard to dangerous falls, dunghills were placed in the streets and not cleared away regularly, and pigs often wandered loose. Animals were slaughtered and butchered along the open stream which ran down through the Market Place, and children used the streets as privies, so it is little wonder that Whitehaven, in common with other eighteenth-century towns, suffered from many epidemic visitations. Brownrigg's Casebook cites an outbreak of epidemic fever in 1737, and in 1743 he himself almost fell victim to another unspecified epidemic, for, as his father-in-law John Spedding wrote to Sir James Lowther:

> April 27 . . . this distemper that is grown more rife than ever . . . we have had very little warm weather . . . this has increased the fever hugely this week, whole familys are seized with it and a great many dye, 2 or 3 in a house.
>
> April 29. More people fall ill every day of this disorder, which makes grievous havoc in some poor familys where the people are crowded into small rooms and have not propper conveniences. Dr Brownrigg was a few days since when one man was lyeing dead, another dying and a third very ill, all in the same little ground room. . . . The Doctor is so harassed he has got a Relapse and is worse this evening than he has been and must be forced to take himself a few days ease to put himself to rights.
>
> May 1. The Doctor has fatigued himself so unreasonably by going amongst his patients on Friday before he was quite well, that he had likely have dyed that night, but by blistering and sweating profusely yesterday he is fine and cool.[36]

[31] Collier and Pearson, *Whitehaven 1600–1800*.

[32] N. Tattersfield, *The forgotten trade*, London, J. Cape, 1991, pp. 326–50.

[33] Brownrigg treated Rhead as a patient. See Case No. 58. There are possibly five versions of this painting. Information from Miss M. E. Burkett.

[34] CRO, Cumulative Rent Book 1743, D/Lons/W5/232 and CRO Census 1762 (copy made in 1762).

[35] Whitehaven Town Book, MSS volume, Jacksonian Collection, Carlisle Library, A242.

[36] CRO, Spedding to Lowther, letters, D/Lons/W.

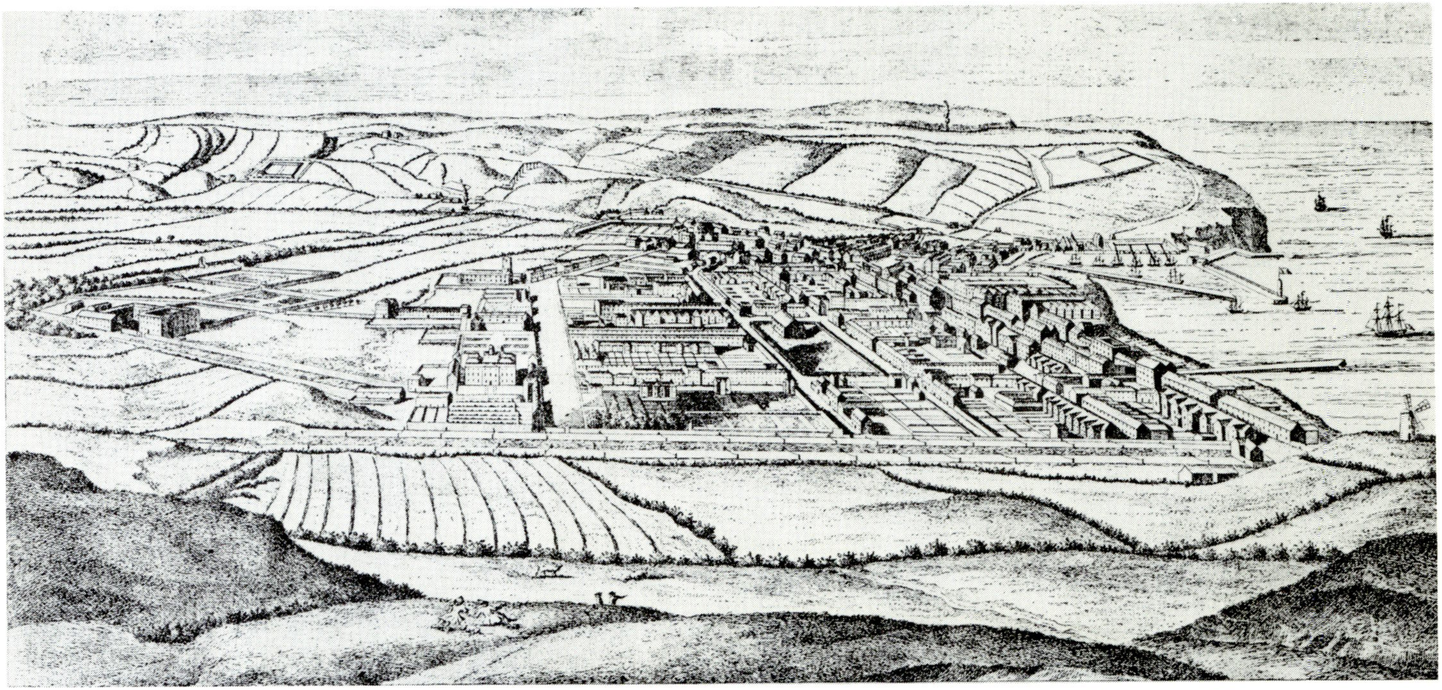

Plate 2: Whitehaven. From an engraving by Richard Parr, based on Matthias Rhead's *Bird's eye view of Whitehaven, 1738.*
(Reproduced with permission of the Whitehaven Museum.)

Epidemics of smallpox, measles and various types of fever occurred in Whitehaven with great frequency, and Brownrigg, in common with medical opinion of the 1730s, related these outbreaks to the prevailing weather, as noted in the final pages of the Casebook. He had great experience with fevers in particular and when, in 1771, a plague in Europe threatened to spread to the towns of Britain, Brownrigg wrote a paper on his own experiences of "Gaol" fever or typhus.[37]

An analysis of the cases in this book reveals the diagnosis and treatment of 127 patients between 1737 and 1742, 69 males and 58 females (see Figure 1) with a range of ages assessed where possible from Brownrigg's information. Of these, there were 28 deaths, the majority occurring between the ages of 20 and 50. All these figures, however, must be accepted as only an analysis of the selective nature of the Casebook and not an indicator of the general age or mortality composition of his entire sum of patients between these dates. While the same caveat must apply, the examination of the social standing of the Casebook's patients is perhaps indicative of the wide range of people he attended. Only 1 labourer (see Figure 2) and 4 servants are representative of the lowest social group, and it is curious that the great number of colliers is not represented at all. It may be, however, that, because of his interest in the gases of the coal mines, Brownrigg kept the colliers' cases of trauma and occupational disease in a separate volume. Thirteen sailors and 13 craftsmen, ranging from blacksmith to plasterer, perhaps represent the second social

Figure 1: Age groups of male and female patients.

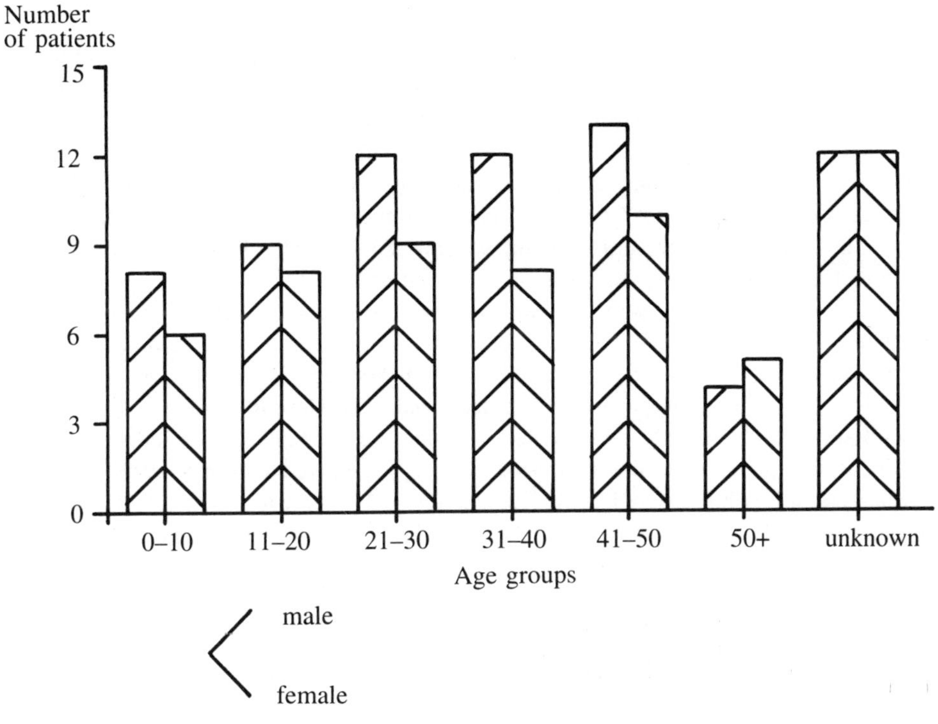

[37] W. Brownrigg, *Considerations on the means of preventing the communication of pestilential contagion and of eradicating it in infected places.*

Figure 2: Known professions of patients.

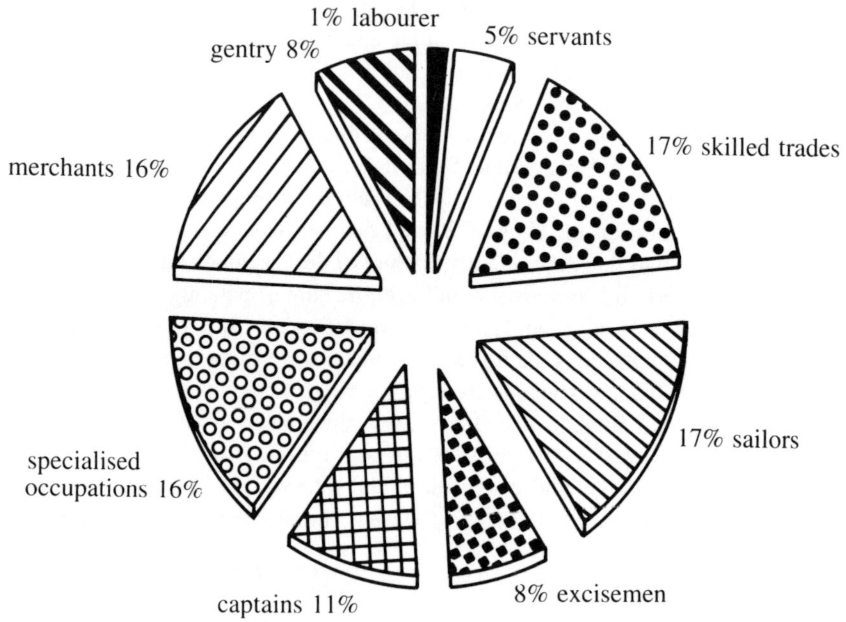

stratum, but most of the remainder would have been able to pay considerable fees for their treatment. These can be divided into Customs officers, ships' captains and 12 people in specialist occupations, ranging from colliery manager and engineer to lawyer and vicar. The social apogee was represented by 12 merchants and 6 landed gentry who would have been able to afford the most expensive cures and prolonged consultations. His most illustrious patient, Sir James Lowther, is not mentioned in the Casebook, but Spedding's letters indicate that he was treated on several occasions by Brownrigg, particularly towards the period of his eventual leg amputation in 1750.[38]

Twenty-five of the Casebook patients were resident outside Whitehaven, and Brownrigg must have travelled to see them at Parton (2 miles), Egremont (6 miles), Workington (9 miles), Cockermouth (14 miles), Hayton (20 miles), Isel (16 miles), Keswick (27 miles), Maryport (15 miles) and Carlisle (40 miles). More distant consultations to Newcastle and the Isle of Man were conducted by letter. His most distinguished patients in the Casebook were Sir Wilfred Lawson from Isel, near Cockermouth,[39] who suffered from haemorrhoids, Master Curwen of the Curwens of Workington Hall, who had rheumatic fever,[40] and Mr. and Mrs. Christian of Unerigg Hall, Maryport.[41] Mrs. Christian had a prolonged consultation with Brownrigg, accompanied by

[38] For his account of the treatment of Sir James Lowther for erysipelas in 1742, see J. V. Beckett, 'Illness and amputation in the case of Sir James Lowther (1673–1755)', *Med. Hist.*, 1980, **24**: 88–92, pp. 89–90.

[39] E. Hughes, *North country life in the eighteenth century; Cumberland and Westmorland 1700–1830*, Oxford University Press, 1965.

[40] Ibid., Workington Hall now stands as a ruin.

[41] The Christian family had strong Isle of Man connections and Mrs. Christian was the grandmother of Fletcher, the *Bounty* mutineer. Unerigg has now been demolished.

correspondence on a great variety of maladies which may have been related to her menopause. An educated woman who was capable of describing her own symptoms in a letter to Dr. Mead in London, she was obviously not satisfied with her own doctor Clementson and had called Brownrigg in for a second opinion. She and her husband received the Brownriggs socially, according to the details of several letters, and Brownrigg himself treated her as an intelligent woman, capable of understanding medical terms relating to her condition as he saw it.

Brownrigg's concept of medicine as illustrated in this Casebook written about 1742 seems conservative and depends on the styles of Sydenham and Boerhaave. Sydenham had introduced therapeutic innovations and particularly promoted the use of quinine as a useful specific in the treatment of fevers and liquid laudanum as a relief from pain. Brownrigg also used these two items for his patients under these circumstances and increased the doses of liquid laudanum greatly in terminal cases (see Case 11 and Case 77). Sydenham studied the nature of disease after the Hippocratic method[42] and made a series of accurate and detailed observations based on the theory of the four constitutions of the body.[43] His practical medical advice included fresh air, exercise on horseback and a moderate diet. Brownrigg held fast to these precepts as essential to treatment (see Case 44 for diet; Case 80 for horseback exercise) and to the belief that fevers changed their characteristics according to the time of year and the nature of the weather (see the final entry in the Casebook).

This mechanistic approach to medicine was also advanced by Boerhaave, Brownrigg's tutor at Leiden. He stated that doctors had to find their own way to diagnosis based on the sound teachings which were available under his tuition. The "Perfect Medical Man" had to have a grounding in mathematics and the natural sciences before advancing to anatomical study of corpses and living animals to examine the structure of the body. To this was then added a study of the body's vital fluids using anatomy, chemistry, hydrostatics and examination by microscope. The normal phenomena of the body were surveyed and the causes of every variation revealed by logical deduction and a personal gathering of details of the effects of diseases and medicines upon the norm. A good doctor had to consult the best writers (see Brownrigg's exhaustive quotes in the section on haemorrhoids) and also examine clinically the external appearance of a patient at his bedside. Boerhaave had implicit confidence in his prescriptions, a careful adherence to diet and physical methods of relief such as footbaths and massage.[44] Haller described Boerhaave as "Communis Europae Praeceptor",[45] which indeed he was, with such a wide range of nationalities as his students. Brownrigg consulted Boerhaave by letter in the case of Robert Gale (Case No. 80) in October 1737, and, despite his ill-health,[46] the master replied with practical advice for treatment and also prescriptions for a pill and a draught. Although the simple microscope had been invented, no case reference is made to its use and Brownrigg employed the naked eye alone in the examination of blood and urine; nor did he use any

[42] J. F. Payne, *Thomas Sydenham*, London, T. F. Unwin, 1900, pp. 222–35.

[43] K. Dewhurst, *Dr Thomas Sydenham (1624–1689)*, London, Wellcome Historical Medical Library, 1966, pp. 140–5.

[44] C. D. O'Malley, *The history of medical education*, Berkeley, University of California Press, 1970, pp. 201–17.

[45] Ibid., p. 211.

[46] Boerhaave was by this time suffering from dyspnoea, which grew worse by April 1738, with anasarca and oedema of the feet and legs.

form of auscultation on his patients. Therapeutics were all important and Brownrigg's were largely herbal-based from the major pharmacopoeias available. Most of the items used would have been common in the medical chests of the period, even Peruvian bark which had been widely adopted in the treatment of a variety of fevers. In cases of extreme pain, he resorted to unspecified anodyne draughts, liquid laudanum and opium. As Whitehaven was a port with contacts in the colonies, Brownrigg employed herbal items from the New World which may have been imported directly, e.g. American bindweed and mulberry, and Virginian snakeweed. From the West Indies, one of the Gale family brought back the Conessi bark to Whitehaven, and although they did not appreciate its therapeutic value, Brownrigg added it to his pharmacy and treated with it patients who were prone to dysentery. Certain disorders are deliberately grouped together in the Casebook and show a similarity in treatment, however, if the initial attempts proved unsuccessful, he did change the prescriptions, particularly in the cases of his wealthier patients. Wines and beers were recommended in many cases as were specific waters, e.g. Scarborough, and Bristol, and physical stimuli and exercise were also advocated. He regarded the cure for the stone without cutting as important; he removed a page from the *Newcastle Courant* on Mrs. Stephens' Medicine for the stone, pasted it into the Casebook and followed it with copious notes on Hartley's and Lobb's expositions. He advocated this cure in the cases of only three patients, perhaps indicating his eventual scepticism of the miracle cure. The lengthy section on haemorrhoids follows the precepts laid down by Boerhaave and can be divided into three sections. Firstly, a list of personal observations and notes from all the major writers on the subject; secondly, the two detailed cases of Thomas Iredale and Brownrigg himself and lastly, a 'Dissertation on Haemorrhoids' which he probably drafted for a publication of his own.

His correspondence section contains copy letters from van Swieten in Holland and several Leiden graduates in Britain who were obviously in agreement with his own philosophy of medicine. This was a normal procedure of the time, and Brownrigg himself passed on advice in letters in the cases of Miss Todd (No. 78) and Miss Cookson (No. 84). One of the local doctors, George Carlyle, even passed on a letter to Brownrigg which he had received from van Swieten on a similar case.[47]

The selective nature of the Casebook does not permit an accurate analysis of the scope of diseases suffered by Brownrigg's patients; however, a classification of identifiable diagnoses (Figure 3) indicates a large proportion of respiratory conditions. These range from the mortality of the Rev. Ashley's daughters from whooping cough (see the section on the Chin-Cough) through the serious chest infection of Carlisle Spedding (No. 57) to persistent coughs, as in the case of Mr Fausett (No. 54). Many types of fever were identified by colourful names—epidemic, inflammatory, infectious, low grade, nervous, hectic—and they beset the population of Whitehaven in epidemics of varying seriousness. In his observations on the weather, Brownrigg related specific fevers to time of year and climate, but drew no definite conclusions from this. In his first year at Whitehaven, "epidemic inflammatory fever" raged in the town and he observed that one-third of the population was affected with what may have been typhus. It had been brought by ship

[47] George Carlyle (1715–1784) practised in Kendal and Carlisle. A MS book of about 220 pages of extracts from Boerhaave's lectures (probably made by his father, William Carlyle) and cases in which Boerhaave was consulted, together with other observations is in the Library of the Royal Society of Medicine.

Figure 3: Identifiable diagnoses

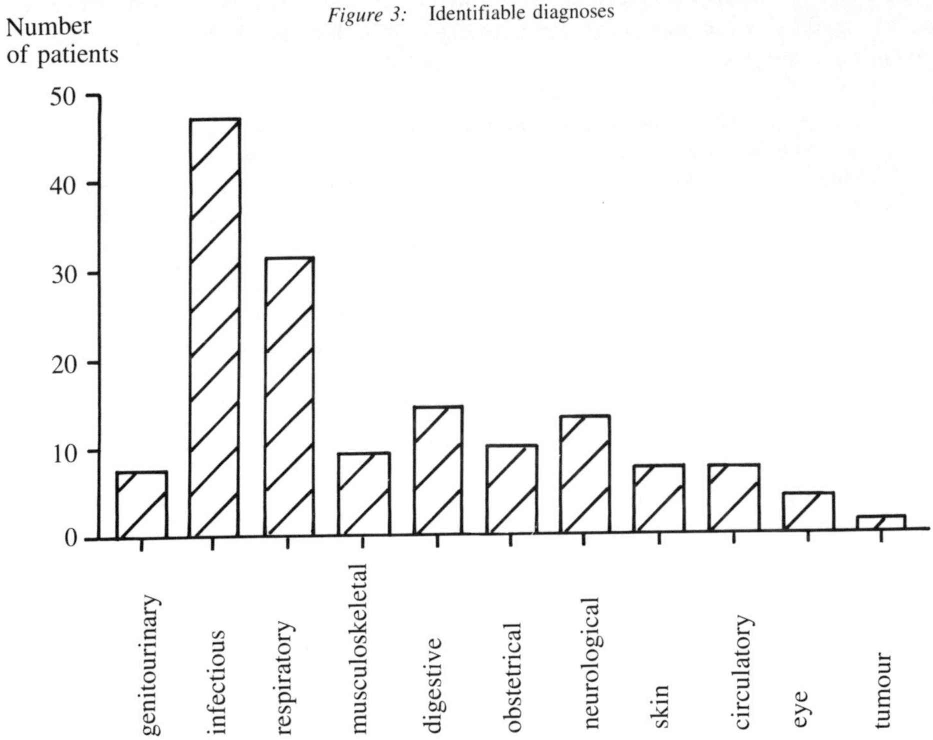

from Dublin, where a similar epidemic raged, and resulted in deaths, particularly among the weak and the young. From five cases of puerperal fever in the Casebook, only Mrs. Drewitt (No. 33) survived, with the others being beyond Brownrigg's help. Mrs. Christian (No. 18) had had an inept midwife and her distress was only eased with increasing doses of liquid laudanum. The death of Mrs. Hudelstone (No. 77) was due to an incompetent delivery, and despite eight days of constant attention, she could only be eased into a state where "her spirit departed in peace" by a massive dose of 24 drops of liquid laudanum and 2 scruples of opium. He attempted to cure his patients, but in some cases it was obvious that the illness was terminal, so, after exhausting his repertoire of therapeutics, he seems to have ceased to treat the patient and only made a note of the subsequent death. This attitude was common in the eighteenth-century doctor, whose patients indeed had less expectation of cure and more familiarity with death than twentieth-century sufferers. If the doctor was deemed to have tried his best, there were no recriminations when he ceased to visit, thus avoiding useless expense to patients and their relatives. Second opinions were often sought and that too was an accepted standard between medical men, although Brownrigg did object to the intervention of a "quack" Amos (Case No. 13).

For almost forty years, William Brownrigg treated the population of Whitehaven with the conservative medicine of his teacher Boerhaave. He may have employed more revolutionary treatments during this period, but the Casebook which follows only covers a short section of his work and should therefore not be used as an indicator of his medical thought throughout his whole career. As a scientist, he was experimental and innovative and his medical work may have later reflected this, for, as his biographer said in Brownrigg's obituary:

> . . . scarcely a family is there of any consideration in that large county which has not on record some instances of the masterly skill, and of the amiable attentions, of Dr Brownrigg. His system of treating disease formed an epoch in the annals of medical practice.[48]

[48] *Gentleman's Magazine*, 1800, p. 387.

THE MEDICAL CASEBOOK OF WILLIAM BROWNRIGG, M.D., F.R.S.

I must essay the path by which to raise myself from the earth and fly victorious on the lips of men.

Virgil, *Georgics* [III. 8–9]

ERYSIPELAS

It was in spring of the year 1738 that the erysipelous fevers first appeared, (a) and they corresponded exactly to those described by Sydenham;[1] (b) the swelling is red, shiny, and confluent with marked pain and heat; on the surface of the swelling there appear at first tiny pustules, which later build up into vesicles. When these vesicles burst, they pour forth a large quantity of thin serous fluid; then if the illness is properly treated, the swelling goes down quickly and the skin heals up. The swelling mostly starts on the forehead; then completely closes the eyes because of swelling of the lids, and from then on it gradually spreads downwards to the lower parts of the face until it finally stops at the neck. In the same fashion it increases in one area and goes down in another; nor are the external features alone involved, for I have often noticed that the tongue becomes very red, (c) dry, smooth and shiny; the nostrils also are often so blocked that it is impossible to breathe through them. This disease is always associated with headache, sleeplessness, thirst and fever, and sometimes delirium and severe malaise. Then if the illness is ineptly treated, it often ends in death. In fact I have heard that many people have perished from the disease during this year, it being widespread everywhere. The blood always appears inflamed. The disease affects adults more than adolescents and men more often than women; it can be said that infants suffer from it now and again. I know that a similar condition may affect parts of the trunk and limbs, but then as well as the inflammatory condition of the humours, there has been another cause which affects the humours in these particular parts, so I know that in a tumour and fistulous abscess-in-ano (d) the adjacent buttocks are affected by an erysipelous swelling and (e) from a light bruising I have noted a tumour of the whole leg.

(a) In the autumn of the same year they were quite common, and with the additional complication of delirium they proved lethal to many who had been badly treated.

(b) Erysipelas differs from the phlegmone, in the fact that the swelling does not pass into suppuration.

(c) I noted this on a woman in her seventies called *Meales* living in Cockermouth, who suffered coincidentally from both coma and delirium, her lungs becoming blocked with phlegm so that her breathing became wheezy. I prescribed nitrous apozema to dilute the phlegm, venesection, clysters, poultices, fotus and vesicatories to the lower legs. With this treatment the inflammation was brought down but she remained very weak for a long time afterwards as a result of her prostration, with severe malaise and vomiting. Eventually however she recovered.

N.B. Before I was consulted the venesection was omitted and heating remedies were used both externally and internally.

(d) As noted in Mr. Pow, a cobbler of this town.

(e) According to Mr. Bewley the pharmacist.[2]

ERYSIPELAS

I do not approve of Sydenham's mixture of spirit of wine and sherry, for experience has taught me that such mixtures increase the heat and inflammation, drive the bad humours

[1] Thomas Sydenham of London.

[2] See Appendix II.

into the brain, worsen headache and bring on delirium. All oily and fatty remedies are also to be avoided for they close the pores of the skin.

In many cases I have tried out an antiphlogistic method with uncommon success. (a) Of course I have carried out venesection two or three times, more or less often depending on the disease and the patient's strength, and to the affected areas I have applied emollient fermentations and poultices made of wheaten bread and milk, sometimes adding Andromachus treacle, and once the inflammation had settled down I have occasionally applied a nutritive ointment to the skin. As internal treatment I have used remedies of nitrous diluents, repeated laxatives made from Glauber's salts in cream of tartar, Manna of Tamarisk and either draughts made from Senna pods or clysters, together with a light diluent diet.

With this treatment I have completely cured Mr. Dan Dixon and Mr. Williamson, ships' captains, and a sailor called Benson,[3] and others.

Erysipelas duplex is 1) Phlegmonoid, with superficial swelling of bright red appearance, with stabbing pain, like the Rosa we call today Rosa Bullata. 2) Oedematous. The swelling is of course fiery, tending to turn yellow, with stabbing pain and rapidly developing gangrene, and I believe that out of the ten phrenetic patients who died, nine perished from this type of disease.
(Boerhaave: Comments in his *Aphorisms*: 380).[4]

Paul of Aegina, Alexander of Tralles and many ancient authors mention, besides phrenitis and peripneumonia, erysipelas involving the brain and lungs, and yet this most useful distinction is often ignored today.

(a) In erysipelas especially, and also in many other conditions when inflammation is present, experience teaches us that scarification of the affected areas, when greatly thickened membranes appear, often causes the whole condition to clear up with amazing speed. Friend [*sic*]. *Opus*. p. 396.[5]

ON THE ERYSIPELOID FEVER 1738

At the beginning of October 1738, the fever was seen by me for the first time, which I, like Dr. Henry Salkeld, call erysipeloid. The illness is very acute and highly dangerous which appears with the following signs and symptoms:

The pulse is generally strong, hard, and rapid. There is thirst, restlessness, and all the other symptoms of acute fever; sometimes the lungs are involved and death soon occurs. There is a feeling of cold from the disturbed brain with frequent shivering attacks, convulsions, delirium and coma; the urine is sometimes pale, and the blood is highly inflamed. Swelling generally spreads over the whole face, and sometimes to the ears, or armpits, and it appears slightly soft and almost liquid; mostly not very red but with marked heat and agonising pain.

An investigation into the nature of the illness: The scalp, periosteum and other membranous parts seem to be the seats of this inflammation; as a result great pain is caused by distension of these areas. The swelling attacks these parts with erysipelas and

[3] William Benson, a mariner who died 10th July 1746 "up the Baltic", aged 46. Buried in St. Nicholas church.

[4] Hermann Boerhaave, *Aphorismi sive de cognoscendis et curandis morbis*, Leiden, J. van der Linden, 1715, no. 380, p. 75.

[5] J. Freind, *Opera omnia*, London, J. Wright, 1733, p. 396.

shows the same appearance. It never goes on to suppuration, but by carrying infected matter into the brain and lungs it rapidly causes death from gangrene of these higher parts, whence it can justly be described as more like erysipelas than the phlegmon.

Question: Is this Boerhaave's Oedematous Erysipelas?

ERYSIPELOID FEVER

This requires very considerable evacuations and an antiphlogistic diet, as will become clear from the following case histories.

On the 2nd October 1738 I was urgently asked to see Widow Troghear's 9-year-old daughter, who was the first patient I saw with this fever.[6] She had already been ill for a week when I was first called in, and one specimen of blood which was withdrawn was of an inflammatory nature. Her pulse was full, hard, and rapid, her breathing was fairly easy, she had thirst, vomiting and great restlessness so that she constantly wanted to move from one place to another; her tongue was white and she had cold shivers once or twice a day, each lasting half an hour; she loudly complained of a terrible pain in her right ear. I let blood twice and this looked very inflamed. I prescribed emulsions and nitrous remedies with a light fluid diet. After three days the vomiting stopped; she complained of pain in her hip joints and numbness of the whole of her left leg; this was followed by spasmodic jerking of the whole leg. Behind the affected ear, there now appeared a soft swelling which appeared to contain fluid, and which I dared not open; then the pain in her ear became less severe, but she then lapsed into a coma and died about the 16th day of her illness.[7]

Second case of erysipelas involving the lungs: On the 6th October I visited William Meales, a blacksmith from Cockermouth who was 45 years old, a robust man and given to drink. Seven or eight days beforehand he had felt an extremely painful swelling in his arm which spread up to his armpit and then went away after 3 or 4 days. His chest was then affected; since the illness was not serious, he was bled once and cardiac remedies were given. On the 5th October, in the evening, the pain in his chest suddenly became very much worse, so he was bled again and this showed signs of inflammation. Next morning I visited him; his pulse was very fast and hard; he had the most terrible pain and burning feeling in the middle of his chest so that his breathing was laboured, shallow and wheezy; with every hour his pulse became weaker and he died the same evening.[8]

Third case, virulent erysipeloid fever: Richard Johnstone, a sailor aged 35, and a robust man who had been ill with a fever for a week. On being summoned on November 5th I noted the following physical signs: rapid though not hard pulse, very severe headaches, restlessness, thirst and insomnia. There was a swelling all over his scalp, most noticeable in the middle of his forehead, which appeared of soft consistency and normal colour. It was at this location that he felt great heat and intolerable pain. I used venesection, cupping glasses, footbath, shaving off his hair, nitrous remedies, purgatives and the application of poultices to his head, nose and forehead. The disease soon left him, but not before the swelling had spread down to his upper jaw and this was where he had the most severe pain.

[6] Ann, the daughter of Elizabeth, a widow. The girl was buried in St. Nicholas church in 1738.

[7] This was probably acute otitis media and mastoiditis with cerebral complications.

[8] The pain and swelling in the arm may have been due to thrombophlebitis. The chest pain could have been either cardiac or respiratory in origin; a myocardial infarction or a pulmonary embolus.

Fourth case: Miss Musgrave from Hayton aged 13, a spotty, delicate girl. She became ill on 13th November, but the illness was not taken seriously as it seemed mild and like a cold, but after a week the fever became worse. She developed a very distressing headache, her appetite completely disappeared, her tongue was coated and dusky in colour. Her face was puffed up into an erysipeloid swelling, which first appeared on her forehead and then spread downward to her nose, upper lips and cheeks. It was attended with great pain, also her urine was pale. Therefore after consultation between myself and Dr. Salkeld she was bled seven times within 6 days and a large quantity was obtained each time, so that the patient often felt faint. On the first occasion the blood had a greenish tinge, and was thick like tallow, and the last time it was markedly inflamed. By using this copious evacuation, local plasters applied to the back of the neck and lower legs, nitrous powders and tartar, with a suitable cooling diet, the disease completely cleared up.

EPIDEMIC INFLAMMATORY FEVER

About June 12th, 1737

1 Isaac Williamson, a sailor.[9] A robust young man of sanguine type, 22 years old and just returned from distant parts. He had a rapid, thin, soft pulse, fever, laboured breathing, frequent vomiting, severe pain in the right side of his back, skin soft, tongue whitish, no appetite, thirst, red urine with a slight sediment. 6 oz. of blood let in the morning which appeared quite satisfactory but just a little inflamed. I was called in the evening.

Twice drew ½ pint of blood from his arm.
A cooling stomachic julep made from Sal Prunella, syrup of lemon and simple distilled water.

June 13th. Pulse stronger and fuller, pain still present but much easier, a cough, thin sputum with a little blood, vomiting still troublesome at times. Sleepy, restless during the night. Bowels rather loose.

Our acid pectoral linctus. A pectoral apozem with honey and 1 pint of water and milk.

June 14th. Cough definitely bad, sputum thicker and copious with a little blood. No appetite, vomiting, restless and irritated at night. Pain almost gone except on coughing.

Repeat the linctus and apozem.

June 15th. Sputum more yellow in colour, less bloody. Profuse sweating mainly around the nose. Bowels looser. Stabbing pain in the side on coughing.

Almond oil 4 drachms; hyssop water 1½ oz; Syrup of balsam 1½ drachms; Spirit of hartshorn 15 drops; Tincture of opium 12 drops: Make a mixture.

June 16th. Slept well, cough still troublesome, also the sputum. Sweating ceased and the other symptoms quite cleared up.

[9] Isaac Williamson may have suffered from lobar pneumonia with pleurisy. He survived to become one of the later Harbour Trustees and a man of some importance in the town.

An antiphlogistic apozem, expectorating, clearing and opening, etc., made from dried burberry root, twitchgrass, foenic, liquorice root, hyssop leaves, coltsfoot, best honey oxymel of squills.

June 17th. Great relief from the apozem. Generally much improved. Recovered quickly.

Take the anodyne draught.

EPIDEMIC INFLAMMATORY FEVER

June 2nd, 1737

2 William Hicks, merchant.[10] Aged 43, robust, of sanguine temperament, obese, used to rich food and wine. After a three-week journey in hot summer weather the following symptoms appeared: shivering attacks, restlessness, insomnia and night sweats. I saw him in the morning. Pulse weak and rather rapid, tongue whitish, sleepy, heaviness throughout his whole body; pain in the lower back and appetite completely absent. His worst affliction was pain in his throat with difficulty in swallowing. Dysuria.

Drew 12 oz of blood from his arm forthwith.

Noon. Blood drawn in the morning appeared rather pale and inflamed, otherwise satisfactory. Urine turbid and dusky with purplish red sediment. Shivering and sweating by turns. Great prostration.

Root of twitchgrass 2 oz; Burberry 2 oz; Tamarisk ½ oz.
Boil for half an hour in spring water to make up 2 pts, adding finally the following items: Liquorice root ½ oz; strain until clear, then add Salt of nitre ½ oz; pure clear honey 1 oz. Make this apozem and take 6 spoonfuls warm every 3 hours. Let his diet be very thin.

June 3rd. At night he got little rest but all the symptoms improved except the sore throat. Bowels moved two or three times. He took a little of the apozem.

Repeat the apozem. A decoction of barley 12 oz; Rose honey 2 oz; Rose water 1 oz; Nitre 2 scruples; Spirit of sulphur and camphor 30 drops.
Gargle with this carefully and warm it first. Drink frequently with a small quantity of juice or any other warmed liquid. Apply warm white bread to the throat.

June 4th. Great difficulty in breathing through the night. Insomnia, some delirium from time to time, and difficulty with swallowing.

Continue to use the prescribed.

June 5th. Same symptoms, but a little better.

Continue to use the prescribed.

[10] One of the merchants who had ships sailing to Virginia and Maryland. He owned a considerable fortune, as he had purchased in England several freehold estates of about £10,000 in value. In Virginia he had also stock, trade interests and property. He became one of the partners in setting up a glasshouse in Whitehaven and a commissioner of the Turnpike Trust. He died on 10th August 1758 and was buried in St. Nicholas church.

June 6th. Still further improvement.

Sal Prunella ½ scruple; Cochineal ½ gr. Take every three hours in chicken broth.

June 7th. Completely recovered.

A SPECIES OF HERPES

May, 1737

3 Nancy Wright, Mrs. Hicks' maid. Vesicles of the size of buckwheat broke out all over her hands; they contained perfectly clear fluid. They were associated with severe itching. After a few days, the skin being very dry and wrinkled, split open and fresh vesicles came out in great numbers for a short time. I cured these by the method described, after liniments of mercury and sulphur and various Hellebore preparations tried but with no success.

Pill Ruff: ½ scruple; Sal Prunella 1 scruple; Venetian turpentine 4 gr. Made up in to 8 pills. Take on alternate days before retiring, up to 5 at a time, and on the following morning drink 2 pts of Scarborough Water.

LEUCOPHLEGMATIC SWELLING

June, 1737

4 Mr. Todd, the carpenter's apprentice. A cachectic youth of 18 with chronic dyspepsia. During recent very hot summer weather he had drunk large amounts of cold fluids. In the space of one night his legs and arm became very swollen with massive oedema. The skin over the affected areas was so stretched as to produce broad red marks. There was only slight fever without itching or noticeable pain.

Sal Prunella ½ oz; Wormwood 16 oz; Cochineal 2 gr; Milk 2 oz. Pound together and divide into 8 doses. Take one every quarter hour with a drink of small beer.

Next day. He repeatedly used large quantities of lotion with powder. Amazingly the swelling became much less, the marks turned to a distinct leaden colour, there was no fever and so all his symptoms had completely disappeared in the interval between one day and the next.[11]

Add crushed grains of any salts and wormwood and continue to use them every 6 hours. Continue for 2 days. Rub arms daily and vigorously evening and morning with a warm, dry cloth of white wool.

OPHTHALMIA

May, 1737

5 Mr. Steel, tide waiter.[12] He was completely cured of an inflammation of the edges of the eyelids, which had persisted for the whole of the preceding winter, by means of the treatment written here.

[11] A strange case. Massive generalised oedema disappearing within 24 hours is most unusual. As is generally the case, there is insufficient clinical evidence to make an accurate diagnosis.

[12] Mr. Henry Steel, Customs officer and Trustee of the Harbour.

Drew 12 oz of blood from his arm.
A soothing electuary 2 oz; Sal Prunella ½ oz; Powdered root of Julep 1 scruple; Rose syrup solution.
Take this electuary with a strong draught of hydrogala milk and water morning and evening. Keep feet in hot water every evening for half an hour.

TRUE OPHTHALMIA

July, 1737

6 Isabel Gunston, a sexagenarian blind in one eye and suffering from ophthalmia in the other. Rapid, shallow pulse; constipation, very down in spirits and with little energy. (Thirst, and no appetite.)[13] The surface of the sound eye was watering and the eyelids were much reddened and inflamed, with burning heat and pain. A week before I was called in, a loaf of bread had fallen down from a height on to her eye, causing slight damage; from that time onwards the condition worsened each day.

A soothing electuary 2 oz; Salt of nitre 3 scruples; Sweet almond oil ½ oz; Rose syrup solution ½ oz. Make up the electuary and take a quantity with chestnut morning and evening every day.

A blood sample was thick and inflamed. She soon recovered with this treatment.

Take St. John's wort 1 peck; Camomile flower 1 peck; Yellow flower of Melilot 1 peck; Red rose flower 2 scruples; head of white poppy 1 scruple.
Boil for 3 or 4 hours diluted in up to 16 oz of water; strain and add 2 scruples of white Vitriol to make a collyrium. Apply the prescription to the affected eye with a moist cloth every 2 hours. Let her diet be light.

N.B. The electuarium was too soft.
Query: Was this the stationary fever?

DISTINCT SMALLPOX

Towards the end of June, 1737

7 Miss Dorothy Nicholson, infant, 17 months old.[14] At first many vesicles full of clear fluid broke out without any particular malaise; after about 6 or 7 days these disappeared; then slight fever developed, and next day there appeared numerous vesicles, surrounded by red maculae, but of a discrete nature. This inflammation proceeded slowly with no real indisposition or high fever, nor did it reach its height until the 7th day of the rash; nor indeed did her face or eyelids swell.[15]

A light diet was indicated. Instead of a medicament there was Sal Prunella simply dissolved in juice and distilled water. The treatment was moderate.

[13] Note added later.
[14] Daughter of Timothy Nicholson, a merchant who traded with Maryland.
[15] We are not told the site of the first eruption of the vesicles. They came out in succeeding crops and systemic disturbance was minimal. Was this chicken pox?

TYPICAL DISTINCT SMALLPOX

About 18th July, 1737

8 Master Hutchinson, plasterer's child, a boy aged 4½.[16] He was seized one evening by an intense feeling of heat, severe pains in his head, vomiting, etc.

> I was called on the third day of the illness. I ordered 3 oz blood let and prescribed the following julep:
> Barley water 3 oz; Milk 3 oz; Crabs eyes 1 scruple; Sal Prunella 1 scruple; Sugar 3 scruples. Take one spoonful every 3 hours.
> I prescribed a moderate regimen.

On the 4th day of the illness vesicles appeared thickly all over his face, yet they remained discrete; his fever was less, however it did not settle completely after the rash erupted.

> 5th day of the illness.
> Sal Prunella 10 gr; Crabs eyes 3 gr; Sugar 5 gr. Crush together and take twice a day in 6 doses.

On the 8th day he reached the crisis; his face and eyelids swelled up, he could no longer see, the eyelid margins were reddened, his fever burned intensely, with restlessness and great tossing about.

> 8th day of the illness.
> Opium and spring water 6 scruples. Sal Prunella 15 gr. Take at 6 in the evening.

Next day, i.e., the ninth day after the onset of symptoms, the inflammation went down, the swelling of the eyelids receded so that by the evening he could see again; the tops of the vesicles on his face became a dusky colour, an indication that they had reached the final stage. Fever much less.

> 9th day of the illness.
> Repeated the paregoric draught.

On the 10th day all the vesicles on his face had completely disappeared.

July, 1737

9 Miss Nicholson,[17] an Irishwoman, suffering from epidemic fever. A single woman of about 20, beautiful, lively, with a good temperament; suffering from hardness of the breasts; very fond of watery food and living a life of idleness. For some time she had been feeling depressed, then during the evening of July 7th she suddenly became very feverish, with vomiting and pain in her head and back. She took nothing but Sal Prunella. On the 9th of July she became confused: 10 oz of blood were removed. Immediately afterwards I was

[16] Brother of Henry Hutchinson, who died of smallpox in 1737 (see later case).

[17] A relative of William Nicholson, a retired sea captain from Whitehaven who had settled in Dublin and had a public house. He had been involved in seeing to a boiler which had been shipped via Dublin for the Newcomen engine at Whitehaven in 1717.

called to see her and found a weak, rapid pulse, deep laboured breathing, whitened tongue, thirst, constipation, urine stringy with slight whitish sediment. Delirium. The blood very slightly inflamed. At 10 in the evening her bowels moved and she became less confused.

> Keep her on a light diet. I prescribed a clyster that she did not allow to be introduced. Black wax water 4 oz; Milk 4 oz; Sal Prunella 2 scruples; Spirit of sulphur and camphor 20 drops; Syrup of violet 6 scruples. Make a julep and take 2 spoonfuls every 2 hours.

The morning of 10th July. She slept 5 hours during the night, all symptoms improved. No fever, skin soft, sweating profusely, no delirium. She complained of heaviness in the head and sore throat.

But at 12 noon the delirium returned, accompanied by a weak pulse. After midday she was better again; in the evening she was again delirious without any fever. Therefore, she was feeling hot and cold by turns, just as Sydenham observed in the Stationary Fever of 1684–5 and succeeding years. And first, as he observed, the patient was quietly delirious, behaving very strangely thereafter.

> Pennyroyal water 1½ oz; Sal Prunella 1 scruple; Opium syrup ½ oz. Take a draught of this at bedtime.
> Root of dried Sea holly ½ oz; husked oats 1 oz; Currant skins 4 oz; Tamarind fruit 3 scruples. Boil in spring water to make up 2 pts. Strain the apozem and add 2 scruples of Nitre. Take 2 spoonfuls every 3 hours.

11th July. Delirium all night. She slept well in the morning; the delirium cleared up and did not return; she soon recovered.

August, 1737

10 Mr. Noblet, from the County of Lancashire, suffering from epidemic inflammatory fever. A robust man of 30, of plethoric build, who had a sudden nosebleed while on a journey. He immersed himself up to the neck in a cold bath and after arriving at his home he indulged in a large drink. That night he suddenly developed a fever.

> Before I was called, Dr. Creighton offered a julep of Sal Prunella and Crabs eyes.

August 1st. 3rd day of the illness. Signs of the disease; weak pulse, burning sensation of heat, rapid shallow respirations, moist skin, swollen face of a livid hue, reddened eyes, severe pain in the back, thirst. He vomited everything he swallowed shortly afterwards, moist white tongue, diarrhoea, urine clear but deep yellow.

> Salt of Wormwood 1½ scruples; Lemon juice 2½ oz; Milky water 5 oz; Spirit of lavender 1 scruple; Lemon syrup 6 scruples.
> Take 3 spoonfuls every 2 hours. Let his diet be light and anti-pyretic.

Afternoon. Acute fever and heat; vomiting; blood was somewhat inflamed. (The blood resembled the fluid in pleurisy.)

> Took 12 oz blood from the arm.

At night, diarrhoea.

Took a paregoric with 12 drops of liquid laudanum.

August 2nd. Slept peacefully at night. Felt hot, thirst, sweating, slight cough, occasional vomiting; occasionally drops of clotted blood came from his nose; pain in back was better; blood less inflamed, urine as before. No response from bowels.

Repeat the julep. Took ½ pt of blood.

August 3rd. No sleep during the night, but slept 4 or 5 hours in the morning. Felt extremely hot, with copious perspiration. Bowels constipated but responded once to a clyster. Blood slightly inflamed.

A phlebotomy was again done and ½ pt of blood drawn from the vein. Take an emollient and relaxing clyster. Drink the cooling apozem. Take 6 spoonfuls of the laxative every 2 hours.

August 4th. Had caught a chill meantime. A very restless night, fever increased, great thirst, very difficult breathing. Thick bloodstained sputum. Pain in side when coughing, hard pulse, blood again inflamed. Further nosebleed, unwisely arrested with vinegar. Deafness.

Took ½ pt of blood. Continued to use the apozem.

August 5th. All symptoms improved, but still a rather hard pulse. Blood less inflamed; occasional stabbing pain in his side. Troublesome cough, laboured breathing, urine thick and bright yellow. Deaf.

Took 6 oz of blood. Continued to use the apozem.

August 6th. Much better.

Continued to use the apozem.

August 7th. Still improving.
August 8th. Now free from pain and fever, but still has a cough.

July, 1737

11 Henry Martin, stonemason,[18] died from intestinal obstruction. A robust man aged 30, who suffered occasionally from colic and always treated himself with large doses of Cardamom seeds. On July 3rd he had his usual pains, and took his usual remedy but without the expected relief, indeed his pain became much worse. An apothecary was therefore summoned on 4th July, who ordered a strong purging enema. After using this, the bowels moved four times. Nevertheless the patient remained in great pain. He was then

[18] The principal master mason in Whitehaven, engaged in building Holy Trinity church and also overseer of the extensions to the harbour. He died on 16th July and was buried in Holy Trinity.

given a purging enema, recommended by Dr. Senhouse,[19] with 1 oz Glauber's Salts and 2½ oz Syrup of Buckthorn which he did not return. On the 5th he prescribed copious amounts of chicken soup and ordered clysters of the same fluid to be administered every 3 hours. The pain persisted and the patient returned only a small part of the clyster fluid. And so, on 6th he ordered an oily mixture and a decoction of plums to drink, but he started to reject everything by the mouth.

July 7th. I was called in about midday. Pulse regular, full and good volume; laboured breathing; skin dry at times, at others pouring sweat. Great thirst, dusky tongue; copious vomit, at first thick greenish material then foul-smelling liquid accompanied by great pain. There was acute pain in the iliac region, somewhat relieved by vomiting; abdomen grossly distended by wind; bowels still closed; urine hardly coloured with slight cloudiness.

Extracted 8 oz blood from the arm.
Milky water 3 oz; Black wax water 3 oz; Weak cinnamon 1 oz; Sal Prunella 2 scruples; Spirit of sulphur and camphor 15 drops; Spirit of lavender 1 scruple; Sugar 3 scruples.
1 full spoonful every hour. He may drink copiously whey or a decoction of plums. The oily mixture may be omitted.

In the evening his blood seemed normal and entirely normal. Rejected matter now yellow. Other symptoms as before.

Cow's milk 8 oz; Olive oil ½ oz; Glauber's Salts 1½ scruples; Rose syrup 3 scruples. Make a clyster.
Mint water 4 oz; Andromachus treacle ½ scruple; Liquid laudanum 50 drops; Opium syrup 1½ scruples. Take half immediately and the remainder after 2 hours.
A blistering plaster was applied to the abdomen made from Andromachus treacle 2 oz; Venetian turpentine 3 scruples, and 10 drops of cloves mixture.

July 8th. In the morning, vomiting stopped at 4 a.m. Great weakness of spirits, weak pulse, insomnia. Abdomen soft, practically no pain. At 10 a.m. returned a clyster mixed with the fluids he had drunk. At 2 p.m. he vomited again.

Mint water 6 oz; Strong cinnamon 1½ oz; Spirit of lavender 40 drops; Liquid laudanum 1½ scruples; Confection of Kermes 1½ scruples. Take 1 spoonful every hour.
At eight in the evening.
Salt of wormwood 1 scruple; Juice of lemon 1½ oz; Mint water 6 oz; Weak cinnamon 1 oz; Pure opium 8 gr; Confection of Kermes 2 scruples.
Make a julep and take 3 spoonfuls every three hours.

July 9th. Slept peacefully during the night, untroubled by sickness. Remained fairly well until evening when he vomited twice a large amount of fluid.

Morning. Continue to use the prescribed julep.
Evening. Salt of Wormwood 1 scruple; Juice of lemon 2 oz; Mint water 6 oz; Strong cinnamon 1 oz; Confection of Kermes 1½ scruples. Take 1 spoonful every hour.
Pure opium 4 gr; Mint water 4 oz; Syrup of cloves 1 scruple; Take half immediately and the rest after 2 hours.

[19] The doctor whose practice Brownrigg joined when he started as a doctor in Whitehaven.

July 10th. Night: restless. Morning: strong and hard pulse; hot; very coated dusky tongue; hard distended abdomen. Thirst less than before. Evening: A little delirium.

Morning: draught taken with 3 gr of opium.
Evening: repeat dose prescribed today.

July 11th. 8 a.m.: again vomited a large quantity of yellowish ingesta. Rapid pulse, now weaker. Dry skin.

Evening: inject an enema of 1 pint of oat juice and 3 scruples of Glauber's Salts.
Keep using the mixture last prescribed.

July 12th. Insomnia and occasional delirium; restless with tossing of the limbs, but without much pain; abdomen sometimes hard, sometimes soft. Pulse faster, weaker and hard. In the afternoon he vomited nearly 6 pints of yellow foul-smelling material, and passed a small amount of extremely offensive stool of a dark colour.

July 13th. Weaker and more restless than ever. In the evening he vomited large amounts of yellow material closely resembling the faecal fluid from his bowel.

July 14th. Symptoms very much more serious. Vomited the same substance two or three times.

July 15th. Vomited the same type of material but in smaller amounts and needing greater effort.

July 16th. Died at 5 a.m. He died a cruel death.

I prescribed on the last days clysters of 1 pint of milk and juice to be injected once or twice daily. Gave a bolus with raw opium. Opium always increases the fever. From the 8th day I used an infusion of mint for a drink and thin juice for food. I told him to remain in bed.

Query: Would mercury have been useful, as successfully used by Dr. Cheselden? Or a clyster from tobaccos made either with mint water or opium and thus correct the putrid humours? Or a cathartic equally strong?[20]

August, 1737[21]

12 Mr. James Lutwidge,[22] died of a stroke. A man in his fifties, of sanguine type, with a large head. Formerly he had been a sailor, but for many years he had suffered from arthritis. He lived an inactive, idle life and indulged in very rich food. Because of constipation he took some laxative medicine which produced diarrhoea, and this responded to binding remedies in about 10 days. Then he became worse and semi-comatose.

By Dr. Hamleton. At first, use was made of a cathartic potion, thereafter a restringent cure.

[20] This man developed acute intestinal obstruction over a period of five or six days. There is no information about the presence or absence of bowel sounds which would have differentiated between paralytic ileus and mechanical obstruction. The latter seems more likely. Today this 30-year-old man would have been referred to a surgeon for urgent operation and relief.

[21] Brownrigg wrote August instead of July.

[22] He was a patient of Dr. Senhouse, Brownrigg's partner, and also a merchant and a member of the locally powerful Lutwidge family. He died on 16th July and was buried in Holy Trinity church.

On the third day of his stupor I was called in and found the following: pulse full, strong, regular and slow; respiration deep and slow; he was sleepy but conscious; he had considerable arthritic pain in his feet and one hand.

> The morning before I was called, Drs. Hamleton and Creighton had prescribed: Cardiac julep; a bolus for the heart; Volatile drops. They applied a blistering plaster to the neck.

I told his relatives that the patient was already lethargic and in danger of a stroke.

> The neck rose well with a blister full of liquid.

The disease however was due more to thick phlegmatic humours obstructing the cerebral vessels than to his arthritis. With the idea of causing their channelling away from the brain, I took the opportunity of prescribing a strong purgative clyster but before it could be prepared he was seized by an epileptic fit, and shortly afterwards he developed a stroke.

> On being called in the afternoon, I prescribed the same. The clyster was bitter: it was not injected.

I could feel no pulse; his limbs were cold; his breathing was deep, laboured and stertorous, with rapid movement of his nostrils with each indrawn breath; his throat was quite swollen; he was incontinent of urine with complete flaccidity of the limbs and with his eyes fixed. As a result all those watching thought that there was already a wake, and that the patient was about to die.

> 1 oz of blood flowed from an incision in a vein.

However, 4 or 5 hours later the pulse could again be felt and after a second epileptic attack he spoke a few rambling words. Therefore:

> Applied blistering plasters on the forearms and shins. Blisters not only rose up, but also split the skin.
> Take 1 spoonful of the cardiac julep every hour. For a drink he should take a mixture of milk, white wine or an emulsion.

So my apoplectic, sometimes speaking a few words or moving his arms and legs a little, with a very weak pulse and bathed in copious cold sweats, was subjected to 2 or 3 epileptic attacks, brought on by either moving about or pain. He was able to swallow satisfactorily until 36 hours later when he died of a convulsion.

EPIDEMIC FEVERS OF THIS CONSTITUTION

Late July, 1737

13 Jane Buntin, a spinster of 22, previously strong and healthy. This woman was suddenly taken ill with an infectious epidemic fever of this type. She sought advice from a quack doctor by the name of Amos. She was bled twice from the arms and given emetics together with volatile spirit and other cooling measures. But she was deteriorating day by day. I was called a week after she had become ill and found: a hard, weak and rapid pulse; extremely

dry skin; tongue coated and dry with a dark film on it; thirst; burning abdominal pain which was unbearable as from torture; she was vomiting and passing very frequent motions, and to crown all she had hysterical spasms. She vomited back both of the sedative draughts I prescribed for her. Next morning I ordered the White Decoction to drink, but she could not swallow it. In the evening I suggested a dose of Conf. Fracastorii. During the evening of the next day, having been urgently entreated to hurry back to the patient because she had very severe diarrhoea, I found she was completely prostrate, with dry skin, fever, jerking of the limbs, a wild expression on her face and inability to utter any articulate speech, but at intervals she wailed aloud in a horrifying fashion.

Amos, who belonged to the same sect[23] as the patient, had applied a poultice to the back of her neck, a little before I was summoned again. When I discerned this, I merely warned him that he should administer a different sedative medicine and then bade him farewell. Amos then applied some leeches to extract blood and ordered rum, saffron and volatile spirits with other vigorous sedative agents. At length the patient, after a huge dose of laudanum, died in a coma, killed off by her disease and the quack.[24]

EPIDEMIC FEVERS OF THIS CONSTITUTION

14 Master Nicholson, a delicate boy aged 9. Towards the end of July he was taken ill with a low continuous fever. Pulse thin, skin generally dry, utterly listless, not particularly thirsty, bowels loose and moving 2 or 3 times a day. He did not feel ill or complain of pain, except for a colicky abdominal pain before moving his bowels. He was lethargic and weary, and lapsed into unconsciousness. His fever was much raised during the night, and in the mornings he had sweating attacks.

He was ill for about 10 or 12 days, and with the use of Sal Prunella and then gentle cathartics he was once more restored to health.

EPIDEMIC FEVERS OF THIS CONSTITUTION

15 John Stockdale's child. A boy of 5 who, in August, had the same type of fever, with the same symptoms, except that he had severe constipation. He had remained poorly for 2 weeks and when I was called in I found him semi-conscious and lethargic. I prescribed a mixture with burdock, crabs eyes and Sal Prunella and in addition the administration of 4 daily enemas of sweetened milk. I forbade the use of his cot for the time being. And when his symptoms were a little improved and his appetite had returned somewhat, I prescribed rhubarb beer for 3 or 4 weeks. Gradually he returned to his former state of health.

August, 1737

16 Richard Tyson, sailor, with a case of dysentery. This man was a crew member of the *Whitehaven Craser*. He was 40 or thereabouts, strong, of moderate eating habits and rather thin. After returning from the island of Eubonia[25] where an epidemic of dysentery was raging, he became ill with this very disease, and had been ill for 4 days when I called in on 2nd August. I found the following signs:

[23] They were probably dissenters.

[24] Clearly this woman had a severe urinary infection and became very dehydrated. Laudanum was not indicated in an already weak and dehydrated patient. When Brownrigg saw that Amos had dealt incompetently with the woman, he had nothing more to do with the case. This attitude was accepted as normal in the eighteenth century.

[25] The Greek island now known as Euboea.

August 2nd. Morning. Slow, strong, but irregular pulse; dry skin; preternatural heat; whitish coated tongue; thirst continous; very severe stabbing pain in the hypogastrium which gradually began to go down to the epigastric region. His frequent motions contained foul-smelling dusky mucous particles, and were mixed with clear mucus. Streaks of blood from time to time with faeces. Blood slightly inflamed.

About noon. Reddish urine with very heavy sediment. After an enema his pulse improved and his pain settled a little; after taking a soothing draught he fell asleep. His pain almost eased, but came back in the morning.

In the morning. Took half a pint of blood from his arm. Keep him constantly in bed. Diet with rice water, rice cooked in milk, and chicken broth ½ pt.
Midday. Cow's milk 10 oz; Mint water 4 oz; Sal Prunella 1 drachm; Diascordium 3 drachms. Make an enema.
Night. Weak cinnamon water 1 oz; Sal Prunella 1 scruple; Liquid laudanum 16 drops; Diascordium 1 drachm. Take this before sleep.

August 3rd. Small amount of thick reddish urine. Pulse steadier and other symptoms and signs the same as yesterday. At first I attempted to treat him with a laxative potion, but he vomited it back half an hour later. Then I ordered a bolus of rhubarb with a decoction of manna and tamarind, ½ oz of each, and cow's milk 6 oz, and spring water 6 oz, to be taken by mouth, of which he vomited the greater part. In the evening he passed many mucous stools. Slight pain.

Morning of 3rd. Tamarind 6 oz; Manna 6 oz; Boil in milk and water until 4 oz. Strain and add ½ drachm rhubarb. Take immediately. Then I prescribed a bolus with 2 scruples rhubarb and a decoction of manna and tamarind.
In the evening. Repeat the narcotic drink.

August 4th. Irregular pulse, pain sedated. He swallowed a potion, a little at a time, which did him good, but in the morning, after the effect was over, he had great weariness and a weak, intermittent and unequal pulse. His pain was settled; there was coldness of the extremities and cold sweats.

4th. Repeat the potion. Repeat the narcotic drink at night.

August 5th. Restful night; once more an intermittent, unequal and weak pulse; urine thick and turbid; pain quite gone; utterly prostrate. At stool he passed small amounts of blackish, fairly offensive faeces. Tenesmus. Skin soft.

5th. Morning. Take a bolus with Confection of Fracastoro 3 scruples; Japan earth 10 grains.
At 2 p.m. Hartshorn powder 3 drachm; Gum acacia 1 drachm; Yolk of egg; Confection of Fracastoro 5 scruples. Mix up and make an enema.
Evening. Repeat the narcotic drink.

August 6th. Generally much improved, except for the pulse. He had moved his bowels only 2 or 3 times in the meantime. Pulse weak, irregular and intermittent.

11 a.m. Repeat the enema.
Evening. Repeat the narcotic drink.

August 7th. Pulse and all signs improved. Practically no pain. Stools small, faecal, dark and offensive.

Powdered hartshorn 2 oz; Gum arabic 3 scruples; Crushed tormentil root 1 oz. Boil in spring water until 3 pts. Strain and add white sugar to sweeten and drink to fortify the potion.
Liquid laudanum (Sydenham's) 2 scruples. Take 20 drops every morning and evening: reduce the dose gradually.

During the next 4 or 5 days, by using these remedies, his bowels completely settled down, his pulse gradually became stronger and more regular. His other symptoms all disappeared, except for the diarrhoea which persisted for some time.

DYSENTERY

August, 1737

17 John Brown, a sailor, a man in his fifties, a crew member of the same ship, was taken ill with the same disease and had the same symptoms except for an irregular pulse. He was much troubled by tenesmus and enormous abdominal swelling, especially towards evening. Now I saw him when he had been ill for 3 weeks. At first I prescribed a laxative medicine, as in the previous case, of which he vomited back the most part. I then ordered an anodyne mixture to stop the diarrhoea and at first he improved on this treatment. But once his pain had settled he declined to follow my advice any longer. After a week I was sent for again and found the patient very weak and listless and tortured by colic. I then prescribed Sydenham's liquid preparation of laudanum, 22 drops to be taken 3 times daily at first, then twice daily. With this remedy alone he recovered within 3 weeks, only his diarrhoea continued for a long time.[26]

N.B.: This pain was so increased by lying down that he avoided going to bed for 3 to 4 weeks.

Towards the end of August, 1737

18 Mrs. Christian, died of puerperal fever.

This woman was 24, tall and of sanguine constitution. She was often affected by hysteria. On the morning of 26th August, without the assistance of a midwife, she gave birth to her first-born, a healthy, lively boy. After delivering the afterbirth she had a copious discharge of pure blood which caused her great anxiety. The lochia then continued to flow quite satisfactorily with occasional remission (until the 8th day[27]).

Day 2. A plaster was applied to her breasts and all went on quite happily until the evening of the next day, when she was seized by violent cold shivers.

Day 3. Next morning she again felt cold with shivering and trembling, which was followed by an intense feeling of heat along with other symptoms of fever. In the afternoon she was anxious. In the evening she was given a laxative enema and was

[26] Three or four sailors from the same ship were affected with the same illness, among them Richard Williamson, whose case history is given below p. 21. Typical of the many seafarers who brought infectious fevers home with them from abroad, these cases were probably bacillary dysentery.

[27] Later addition.

immediately affected by abdominal colic. Her bowels moved once, then by treating her with 17 drops of liquid laudanum, the colic settled down and she had a good night's rest.

An enema made from an emollient decoction of syrup of buckthorn 1 oz: Then 17 drops of liquid laudanum.

Day 4. Morning. Pulse rather hard, full and rapid; the artery full and slowly contracting; breathing freely; tongue whitish coated, moist; troublesome thirst; profuse sweating; rather sleepy.

Afternoon. Skin drier; fever higher; increase in thirst.

Evening. Fever very high; respiration rapid and laboured, with a marked feeling of burning pain in the chest. There was a slight cough inhibited by acute pain while coughing; very severe headache; dry skin; burning, stabbing pain on micturition. Borborygmi and dysuria.

Diet should be barley water and similar thin, non-spiritous liquids. Crabs eyes 1 scruple; Sal Prunella 1 scruple; Sugar 10 gr; pulverise and take 8 hourly.
In the evening I made an injection of enema made from milk and sugar. Then I let 1 oz of blood. Then 14 drops of liquid laudanum.

Bled 1 oz from her arm. This was as good as possible. About midnight the fever had settled a little; there was slight dampness of the skin. I treated her with 15 drops of liquid laudanum and with this she obtained some beneficial rest.

Day 5. Morning. Fever down; respiration satisfactory; slight cough causing pain and much less headache; thick, offensive perspiration; urine thick and turbid with a considerable dark coloured sediment; scattered stabbing pain.

Afternoon. Bowels moved. 3 feverish attacks, but they were not severe.

Fennel root 4 oz; Parsley 4 oz; Liquorice 1 ½ oz; Currants 4 oz. Make up a decoction in water to 3 pts. and drink freely. Apply a resin plaster to the abdomen. Cold quince seed 1 oz; Blanched sweet almonds 1 oz; Barley water 2 pts; Sal Prunella 3 scruples; Syrup of marshmallow 1 ½ oz. Make an emulsion and drink freely. Take the powders as before.

Day 6. Bowels moved twice. Afternoon, fever exacerbated; headache, but not so severe as before. No sleep all night; great restlessness; skin even drier.

In the evening administered: Liquid laudanum 10 drops; Spirit of hartshorn 15 drops; mix in julep flower 3 spoonfuls.
At 10 p.m. I prescribed 10 drops of liquid laudanum.
Continue to use yesterday's prescription.

Day 7. Morning. Moist skin; hot and moderate fever; skin beginning to break out into a rash and flaking. She then developed hardness and swelling first in the thighs, then the arms, then the whole trunk, breasts and up to the armpits. This is a type of illness which women call Felon. No increase in fever; hardly any headache; no sleep at night.

Fennel root 3 oz; Asparagus root 3 oz; Liquorice 1 oz; Sal Prunella 1 ½ scruples; Currants 4 oz; Root of dried sea holly 3 scruples. Boil in spring water to 3 pts. Drink freely.

Powdered shell 10 gr; Sal Prunella 10 gr. Make a powder: take by any means every 6 hours.

Day 8. Moist skin; some heat and fever with a normal, but slightly faster pulse. At night she slept, so I was told, for 3 or 4 hours.

Headache plaster 2 parts; blistering plaster 1 part. Make these plasters and apply 2 to the feet.

Days 9 and 10. She remained about the same for the next 2 days except that she hardly slept at all at night.

Days 11 and 12. Hard, dry skin; stabbing hot flushes; regular pulse; tongue now black; unquenchable thirst; insomnia but no headache. The urine, until now thickened with a sediment, became pale. No matter which way she lay in bed localized pain immediately seized her and she became listless and extremely restless.

Day 11. I applied plasters of Dr. Clementson, and also for the stabbing pain, used rubbings. Emollient enemas had been administered almost daily.

Blood taken from her arm on the 12th day was rather inflamed. On the same day, at 2 p.m. she got out of bed. After lying down again she became unconscious, her pulse rate could not be felt and at 9 p.m., following terrible abdominal convulsions, she died. After death widespread purplish marks occurred and a few hours later the corpse stank horribly.

N.B.: On the 9th or 10th day, small vesicles full of clear fluid broke out all over her body.

N.B.: After this patient's death, the suspicion arose that the midwife, who was overconfident and inexperienced, had carried out her duties very badly. This was shown by the fact that she observed severe pain persistently sited in the right side of the hypogastrium which she, through excessive caution, concealed from me. Therefore possibly some part of the placenta or a bloodclot had been retained in the uterus.[28]

Towards mid August, 1737

19 Frances Elliot. Died of epidemic puerperal fever. This woman was lying in after the birth of her first child. A robust, previously fit woman who had a perfectly normal delivery of a healthy baby girl. The lochia continued to flow nicely for 15 or 16 days, nor was there any problem with the flow of breast milk.

4th day after delivery. She took a fever which the midwife stated was not dangerous, but she was prescribed a sleeping draught, etc., for a hysterical upset.

14th day. I found the following phenomena: weak, regular, fast pulse; prickly heat; skin at times hard and dry, at other times profusely sweating; breathing laboured and rapid; slight cough; tongue blackish and coated; great thirst; vomiting; pains in the breasts and in many other areas; urine reddish with much sediment; pain and swelling of one leg so that

[28] One of five out of six cases of puerperal fever and post-natal complications who died. They were all aged 30 or younger, several with other young children. These tragic deaths could have been prevented if the midwives had practised the most elementary hygiene, and if antibiotics, available today, had been used. An example of the limitations in clinical diagnosis and management of patients in the pre-bacteriological era.

she could not move it; deafness; eyes fixed and staring; semi-conscious; frequent sobbing; bowels constipated; rapid fluttering of the nostrils.

For a suppository: 3 or 4 raisins soaked in oil and inserted in the anus.
Twitchgrass root 2 oz; Fennel root 2 oz; Sea holly root ½ oz; Liquorice root 1 oz; Crushed currants 3 oz; Pure nitre 3 scruples. Mix with spring water up to 2 pts. Having made this apozem take 3 spoonfuls every 3 hours.

15th day. Bowels moved; otherwise as before.
(Morning. Fever rather less, but then she was seized by rigors and cold shivers alternating with bouts of fever. After 10 there was some sweating but this did not relieve her.)

Continue to use apozem.

16th day. In response to the loud entreaties of the midwife and bystanders, I prescribed an anodyne draught which made her constipated. During the next few days two plasters were applied to her head and feet, and a plaster to the back of her neck. However this did little to improve her symptoms. Furthermore, she now developed delirium and complete collapse, her pulse became extremely weak and disordered, and finally about the 24th day after delivery she died.

August, 1737

20 Archibald Mackdonald,[29] a Scotsman, cured of epidemic fever. This man was 33 and earned his living by preparing flax. He was of good temperament and hard to purge.

On the 2nd July he suddenly developed a fever.

August 2nd. Dr. Hamleton saw him; venesection and an enema with a julep, bolus, and drops for headache were ordered.

August 6th. I was called in. Pulse full, strong and rapid with slow contraction and dilation; severe thirst; tongue coated and dusky but moist; sweating and dryness of the skin by turns; copious urine, reddish and clear; troublesome dysuria; terrible headache so that he could not sit upright.

Twitchgrass root 2 oz; Burdock root 2 oz; Asparagus root 2 oz; Liquorice 2½ oz; Tamarind 6 scruples; Cream of tartar 2 scruples; Currants 3 oz; Soak in spring water and make up to 2 pts. Strain and take 6 spoonfuls every 2 hours.

August 7th. No change. Only one motion as a result of the enema.

Repeat the apozem as before. Inject a laxative enema. Shave off the hair.

August 8th. Persistent severe headache in the left side of the head, travelling towards the ear, which caused twitching of the zygomatic muscle on that side. Dry skin and increased heat, otherwise no change.

[29] A flax worker, probably employed by James Hogarth, a linen manufacturer. Hogarth donated his house, 107 Queen Street, as the first Whitehaven Dispensary.

Confection of hops 1½ oz; Dog rose hips 6 scruples; Cream of tartar 2 scruples; Sal Prunella 2 scruples; Lemon juice of sufficient amount to make up an electuary. Take as prescribed with a smaller dose as required.
Drew 8 oz of blood from the arm.

Evening. The small amount of blood drawn in the morning was too little different from normal, so I repeated the venesection; pulse less forceful; tongue now truly coated and black, really dry and covered with sticky mucus: his other symptoms became more acute and were accompanied by a stabbing pain all over his skin. While trying to sit on a chair he was seized by violent epileptic tremors. After this, the fever became less and he regained all his senses intact. So for a change I thought it necessary to use a remedy of prime efficacy.

Evening. Apply an epispastic on the head. Inject an enema of milk, water, oil and sugar syrup. Cream of tartar 2 scruples; Tamarind fruit 1 oz. Boil for half-an-hour in 4 oz. spring water adding to the boiled-down concoction 1 oz of manna. Take the potion at once.

August 9th. Fever and headache much less. Fifteen times or more at stool during the night, and tenesmus, severe dysuria, with pain in the urethra.

Drink copiously of the emulsion. Take the electuary prescribed yesterday.

August 10th. Slept well all night. Weak but full pulse; moderately raised febrile heat; headache nearly gone; great thirst.

Evening. Burning heat and dryness of skin; pulse stronger.

Repeat the liquid solution adding ½ oz tamarind. In the afternoon, if the bowels do not respond, inject a laxative enema until there is a copious evacuation.

August 11th. Good night's rest; weak but otherwise normal pulse; fever heat almost gone; sweating; still unquenchable thirst.

Repeat the potion and if the bowel has not moved after 2 hours, repeat after 3 hours. Cream of tartar 3 scruples; Manna 1 oz. Make a concoction in 1 pt. spring water. Take the draught as soon as possible until there is an evacuation.

August 12th. Same as yesterday; weary and great prostration; thick, copious perspiration.

Elixir of vitriol ½ oz: Take 5 drops every hour in a glass of Bristol water. Inject a 2 oz enema until there is an evacuation.

August 13th. Pulse stronger and quite slow; great thirst; tongue still black; profuse sweating; semi-conscious; dizzy on the slightest movement.

N.B.: Only today he began to take the drops. In the evening the enema was given until there was an evacuation.

August 14th. Slept deeply all night; pulse as before; thirst not quite so severe; less sweating.

1 oz of an enema. Take the prescribed drops.

August 15th. No sweating or thirst, and other symptoms have improved. He continued with exacerbations of fever for one or two nights. The exudate and black coating on his tongue cleared up and he gradually recovered his strength and appetite.

He continued to take the drops and the laxative enema falsely applied for a congenital condition.

August, 1737

21 Barbara Roddery. Epidemic fever. A woman about 30 and subject to hysterical attacks.

August 12th. I was called in today; by this time she had been suffering from a fever for 10 days. Blood drawn from her arm on two occasions was indicative of inflammation. She has had continuous fever with exacerbations during the evening; cough; vomiting; passing of wind; thirst; moist whitish tongue; stringy urine with heavy sediment. Pain in the hypochondriac region and insomnia. Treatment with the apozem produced diarrhoea and all her symptoms disappeared except for a generalised severe abdominal pain which had troubled her previously.

Fresh burdock root 3 oz; Dried root of sea holly 1½ oz; Liquorice root 1 oz; Crushed currants 2 oz; Tamarind fruit ½ oz; Pure nitre ½ oz. Boil for half-an-hour in 2 pts spring water. Take 6 lukewarm spoonfuls every 3 hours.

September, 1737

22 Mr. Richard Williamson[30] cured of inflammatory epidemic fever. A ship's captain about 35 years old, a man of good temperament. He took ill with a fever on 27th September while at sea. After reaching port on 29th Dr. Hamilton bled him from the arm and prescribed a cough linctus with an emulsion and injected a laxative enema. The next day, venesection was repeated and he ordered powders with Sal Prunella, etc., but in the meantime his condition deteriorated and I was called in about midday.

4th day of illness. Pulse feeble, weak and a little faster than normal; intense heat, skin sometimes dry, at other times bathed in sweat; breathing rapid and laboured; slight cough with thin sputum mixed now and again with streaks of blood; moderate thirst; tongue white, scurfy and moist; thick turbid urine of yellowish-white colour. Generalised severe pain round the sides of his chest; very troublesome headache; feeling very ill; bowels constipated; considerable prostration.

Fresh fennel root 2 oz; Fresh twitchgrass root 2 oz; Fresh burdock root 3 oz; Fresh liquorice root 1½ oz; Crushed currants 2 oz. Boil in 32 oz spring water. Take 6 lukewarm glasses of this substance, strained, every alternate hour. For the ordinary decoction, make up with: Cream of tartar ½ oz. Boil in 12 oz spring water, strain and add a lenitive electuary. Make an enema and inject at night.

5th day of illness. After a second dose of the apozem he suddenly felt the chest pain become less severe, and afterwards it went away completely. Slept well during the night.

[30] Died 16th April 1757 aged 56, and was buried at St. Nicholas church.

Next morning he passed three liquid stools following an enema. Copious thick sweat; urine more stringy with very thin sediment. 6 or 7 stools were produced by the apozem. Headache much better. His pain and malaise improved completely and only his cough still troubled him.

> Tamarind fruit 1 ½ oz; Cream of tartar ½ oz; Oatmeal 1 oz. Boil in 32 oz water and add to complete, 10 oz manna. Take 4 oz lukewarm every half hour. From then on persist in taking the apozem first prescribed.

6th day of illness. Moderate thick perspiration and a cough, otherwise quite well.

> Repeat the purgative apozem, to be taken this morning as before.

7th day of illness. So as to relieve the cough and to bring about a complete cure of his illness, I prescribed an electuarium with the desired result.

> Powdered myrrh 3 scruples; Cream of tartar 3 scruples; Powdered nitre 2 scruples; Sweet almond oil 6 scruples; Lenitive electuary 2 oz; Balsamic syrup ½ scruple; Spirit of lavender ½ scruple. Take 4 times a day.

The month of October, 1737

23 Rodgers, a sailor of 22, a robust agile youth of fine bodily temperament. While in dock in Dublin harbour he was seized by an infectious fever, with pain in his side; breathlessness; cough; headache and diarrhoea. Only hot juleps to cause sweating and bind the intestines were prescribed, and whey to drink.

6th day of illness. Evening. A bounding, hard pulse; breathing slow but quite laboured, requiring an effort with his whole chest; cough; great prostration; occasional sweating; bowels now a little constipated; tongue moist; normal colour; persistent pain in the side; great weakness.

> Take 10 oz blood from the arm. His diet should be a mixture of milk and juice, suitably diluted. Almond oil 2 oz; 6 drops of violet. Mix together and add, honey 2 oz; Syrup of red poppy 1 oz; Lavender spirit ½ scruple. Take 1 spoonful for 3 hours and afterwards 3 spoonfuls of the mixture.

7th day of illness. Blood inflamed, with a large quantity of serum.

8th day of illness. Following night, hardly any sleep; abdomen tense; pain in his side and breathlessness still present; thick sputum, sometimes dirty, sometimes clear; pulse slow and forceful.

> Spring water 5 oz; Hyssop water 5 oz; Dog rose 1 ½ oz; Nitre 3 scruples; Tincture of saffron 3 scruples; Elderflower 3 oz. Make a mixture.

9th day of illness. Symptoms much improved. He got out of bed and improves daily.

October, 1737

24 Mrs. Hicks' maid, Molly. A pretty girl of about 22 years old, liable to hysterical disorder and of loose fibre. She had had a menstrual loss for 3 weeks.

Day 1 of the illness. Evening. Small, rapid pulse; hot febrile skin; not particularly oppressive thirst; very severe headache. Skin moist, tongue moist and of normal colour. Breathing satisfactory. She was beginning to have shivering and vomiting.

> Took ½ pt of blood from her arm. Hyssop water 1 ½ oz; Sal Prunella 2 scruples; Tincture of saffron ½ scruple; Sugar 3 scruples; Lemon 3 scruples; Elderflower 3 scruples. Take this draught at bedtime.

Day 2. Blood inflamed and with a large amount of serum. Sleepless night. Rather weak pulse; skin soft; moderate fever; thick, turbid urine looking like whey, with extensive cloudy areas of the same colour.

> Ingredients of this concoction for the chest. Make up 32 oz. Tamarind fruit 2 oz; Pure nitre 3 scruples. Boil in water to 32 oz. Strain and add elderflower 1 oz. Take 6 spoonfuls of this apozem every 3 hours, lukewarm.

Day 3 and later. She took some laxative apozem, but on getting out of bed brought most of it up and vomited everything she swallowed that day and the next. The bowels moved twice in response to treatment with the apozem. Meanwhile she was troubled by headache and general malaise; her tongue became whitish but moist and she became utterly exhausted with pallor of the cheeks and lips. The fever cleared up within 6 days, however she remained weak and very listless with dizziness and malaise from time to time.

> Tamarind fruit 1 ½ oz; Cream of tartar ½ oz. Boil in 16 oz spring water, strain and add 1 oz manna. Take 4 oz of the apozem immediately then every half hour, lukewarm.

October 5th, 1737

25 Mrs. Ferin[31] of Duke Street, suffering from rheumatism. This patient had been ill for a week, with fever and thirst and then she was suddenly attacked by very severe pain, tearing in nature and involving all her limbs so that she could not move her arms nor even one finger. Then came swelling which did a little relieve the pain. Her limbs began to go down and then she again suffered pain of the greatest severity, spreading from time to time to her head and chest. This woman was about 35 years old, she had had very many children and at this time was suckling a five-month-old baby.

> Extracted up to ½ pt of blood from her arm.

Her blood showed inflammation, with a large quantity of thick serum. Treatment with purgatives produced 8 bowel motions and the pains improved with these pills.

> Calomel 10 gr; Guaiacum gum 15 gr; Peruvian balsam 3 drops; Balsam syrup; make up a pill as directed.

Next day. She improved considerably. Her bowels responded well to the purgatives. After a gap of two days the purgatives were repeated, but she felt very weak. Towards evening her chest was affected by pain of the greatest severity which was not relieved in the slightest by

[31] Mrs. Eleutheria Ferin, who was wealthy enough to subscribe £100 towards the harbour works in 1743.

the pills. After the purgatives and pills had been repeated for four more days, all the pain settled down, except for one area only, the scapula.

> Senna leaves 2 scruples; Tamarind 1 oz; Cream of tartar 2 scruples; Manna 3 oz. Make a decoction in spring water and take the potion.
> Matthew's Pill: Venetian soap 10 gr; Peruvian balsam 3 drops. Make up 4 pills. Take one when going to bed, after the purgative potion has worked. Diet should be of milk, juice of stewed apples and similar items.

October 19th. As an epidemic fever of an inflammatory nature was raging everywhere, it attacked our patient already weakened by her previous illness. This fever was fairly acute and marked by a headache, slight cough and troublesome catarrh, so that thin clear fluid poured from her mouth like a river. She was also troubled by her great thirst, but it was especially noticeable that the rheumatism was troubling her not in the least, except for the pain the patient felt in her scapula, as was the case before the fever started. Four days later she suffered shivers, fierce and cold, although she could feel burning heat in her limbs. Her fever still remained and her skin felt hot to the touch in several inflamed areas.

October 25th.[32] Next day all these symptoms disappeared along with the fever, but pain tortured the unhappy woman again. Severe rheumatic pains wracked her; she was coughing up thick mucus in large amounts. Her appetite was reduced to almost nothing so that her diet consisted only of whey. Therefore I prescribed the apozem.

> October 25th. Root of fresh burberry 4 drachms; Root of fennel 1½ oz; Root of common parsley 1½ oz; Root of liquorice 1 oz; Pounded currants 2 oz; Salted nitre 5 scruples; Boil for half-an-hour in spring water to the amount of 32 oz. Take 3 spoonfuls every 2 hours.

November 1st. The production of mucous sputum has continued until now, she has a very weak stomach and her bowels are constipated. Her pain is much less and so I prescribed some pills.

> Gum ammoniac 3 scruples; Gum sagapenum 3 scruples; make an electuary. Liquorice extract 3 scruples; Pill Ruffus 1 scruple; Aniseed oil 12 drops; Balsam of copaiba, which should be mixed with 1 scruple of liquid to make up 12 pills. Take 2 hourly every day.

The weakness of the limbs lasted a long time, but the pain went away together with her other symptoms.

October 10th, 1737

26 Anthony Barras, a fisherman. This man in his fifties was of good bodily temperament and had been suffering from very severe headaches for three weeks. The pain, which affected all parts of his head, but especially the forehead, tortured him without remission. There was no swelling or redness. Pulse very weak, slow and small; cold all over his body; bowels constipated. Mr. Creighton, the night before I was called in, had applied a plaster to the back of his neck.

[32] This following section was inserted after the case of Anthony Barras (No. 26).

Pill Ruffus 1 scruple; Guaiacum gum 1 scruple; Venetian soap 3 scruples; Venetian turpentine. Make up a pill and take 3-hourly every day. Rub the head with a dry, warm cloth. Keep the feet warm in water.

14th. The pain had improved not a whit. Bowels still constipated.

Pill Ruffus ½ scruple; Calomel 10gr; Sal Prunella 10 gr; Peruvian balsam. Make a pill and take 4-hourly at bedtime and the remainder in the morning. Shave the head and apply a blistering plaster.

15th. He took some pills in the evening which made him feel ill and the following morning produced two offensive soft, yellow stools. As I was unable by any lawful means to help him, I stopped seeing him. Thereafter he dragged out a most miserable existence, enduring the most dreadful torments (I heard) often troubled by spasms, and he died about 29th October.
N.B.[33] His wife told me he had taken a vomiting dose from the roots of the white lily, then he was seized by paralysis of one side, delirium, and was firstly shaken by violent convulsions, then went into a coma, and death came to this poor man after another day.[34]

August/September, 1737

27 Baby, son of Henry Hutchinson the plasterer,[35] a case of confluent smallpox. This infant was a year old when I was called in because he had been ill with confluent smallpox for 3 weeks, and for the whole time his bowels had been constipated.

Symptoms. Fever; very deep sores all round his face; eyelids closed; breathing rapid and laboured; convulsive paroxysms of the whole body; frequent convulsions affecting the abdomen and around the mouth. His right hand went into rigid spasm, then his left hand and finally his feet. Treatment with the apozem produced one or two green motions daily. For another three weeks this poor baby continued to suffer, hardly swallowing anything. During his last few days, blood flowed freely from the eroded blood vessels of his forehead, then he died a miserable death.

Tamarind fruit 6 scruples; Cream of tartar 3 scruples; Pearl barley 3 oz; Liquorice root 3 scruples. Boil in spring water to the amount of 24 oz, add afterwards Manna 1 oz. To the collation add 3 oz honey. Having made this apozem, take 1 spoonful every hour during the day until the stomach is loosened.
I prescribed from then Manna, by which he was loosened 5 or 6 times, but without alleviation.

August/September, 1737

28 Master Charles Dean,[36] a boy of 5 years old, of thick, fat constitution.

3rd day of illness. Tiny densely crowded vesicles broke out with reddened areas between them. Persistent fever; frequent colic attacks causing diarrhoea and spreading to the loins. In the following days the thickly spread pustules on the face became raised and some became umbilicated. Larger pustules were present elsewhere on his body. Delirious.

[33] Inserted as a separate footnote under the list of prescriptions.
[34] The history suggests a cerebral tumour.
[35] The family lived in Irish Street. Baby died 5th September 1737 and was buried at St. Nicholas church.
[36] Son of Joseph Dean, the Tide Surveyor (a Customs post) of Whitehaven port.

His diet should be apples boiled in tea, toasted bread with butter, milk and watery beer.

6th day. Fever has almost gone. Eyelids so swollen he cannot see.

After the sixth day he took a soothing draught every night with Sal Prunella. His face was anointed with almond oil, from which he received great relief.

7th day. Copious stools.

8th day. Huge vesicles filled with clear liquid have formed on his limbs and trunk; the areas between the vesicles on the face are red; but elsewhere on his body they are white with red edges. Fever settling; swelling of the face much less.

9th day. Fluid in the facial vesicles almost white, although clear elsewhere.

10th day. Delirious and very restless. The fluid from some vesicles on his legs and thighs is dark and flowing freely. There are still many vesicles with this fluid. Great weakness. Feeling cold.

11th day. Same symptoms. One or two bowel movements.

Day 10 and 12 of the illness I permitted a concoction of Canary wine to be drunk freely, and also the following days.

Next few days. Bowels moving 2 or 3 times daily; symptoms gradually subsiding. After 2 weeks he was able to get up and walk about again.

Towards the end of September, 1737

29 William Lees, blacksmith.[37] A case of rheumatism and pulmonary abscess. This man was about 45, he was formerly obese but is now emaciated. He was used to hard physical work and was a drunkard with an intemperate way of life. For several years he had suffered from rheumatism, for which he tried many different remedies, especially laxatives.

Signs of illness: Severe chest pain so that he can hardly breathe or speak. He feels this pain beneath the sternum, with a hissing and crackling noise in the middle of the chest around the joints where the ribs meet the sternum. This noise can be heard by people near him. He has a hard oedematic swelling the size of a hen's egg on top of the sternum which first appeared three months ago. He has intolerable sciatic pain in his right thigh, and other pains spread over his whole body. On his left knee he has two hot inflammatory swellings, one below and one above the joint on the medial side. There is also a dropsical swelling of the leg. Fever, thirst and cough present.

Took 12 oz of blood.

Blood taken from his arm was thick and inflamed. A large amount of turbid, whitish serum.

Gum of Opopanax 2 scruples; Ammoniac gum 2 scruples; Myrrh gum 2 scruples; Venetian soap ½ oz; Camphor ½ scruple; Oil of nutmeg 20 drops; Venetian turpentine 2

[37] He was described in the burial register of Holy Trinity church as a Nailer.

scruples. Make up to 10 pills and take one four times daily. Up to 4 oz of a strong decoction of Guaiacum after each dose.
Diet should be a mixture of milk, whey, juice, apples and tisane. The leg was rubbed with linen cloths.

Next day. Chest pain rather less. Pulse weak and of small volume.

The treatment was repeated and ½ pt of blood drawn.

Blood not so inflamed as it was yesterday with copious thick sputum.

At night a blistering ointment was applied to the neck. Liniment to be rubbed on his chest.
Applied a blister to the upper thigh.

Three or four days later, by using bread, milk and butter poultices, the two inflamed swellings were brought to suppurate, and when opened with a surgical scalpel, 1 pint of pure pus was obtained. As the sciatic and chest pain still remained, the venesection was repeated twice and a vesicatory was applied to the thigh.

Took blood from the arm and from a second place on alternate days.

Blood inflamed as before. The tearing sciatic pain ceased after the application of the vesicatory and some dull pain remained.

Pill of styrax 8 gr; Venetian soap ½ scruple. Make the pill and take as prescribed.
After all the pills were taken I prescribed the following electuary. As it was too moist I made this addition:
Natural turpentine ½ oz; yolk of an egg. Mix well and add Guaiacum gum 3 scruples; Myrrh 3 scruples; Liquorice extract 6 scruples; Honey 3½ oz; Camphor 1½ scruples.
Take as much as a nutmeg twice daily.

(N.B. After using the vesicatory there was no dysuria because of taking the pills.)

Bowels no longer constipated because of the pills, and as his nights were sleepless and wearisome, I was obliged to prescribe pain-killing tablets quite often, as a result of which the pain was wonderfully relieved.

His inflammatory abscesses were almost healed and his pain very much better, although he was quite prostrate with weakness.

About October 22nd his skin and the white of his eyes became yellow, fever rose up and whole pieces of lung mixed with blood were being coughed up. On October 24th he died, asphyxiated by purulent material.[38]

[38] The emaciated condition of this man, together with his chronic alcoholism (usually associated with poor diet and nutrition), the swelling on the sternum and left knee which produced large quantities of pus, and the expectorated blood-stained lung tissue, all strongly suggest chronic tuberculosis.

October, 1737

30 Master How[39] wasting from measles and from a consequent fever last spring. This boy was 5½ and was very delicate as he had been weakened by smallpox. He had been ill for a week with epidemic inflammatory fever without any really acute symptoms. He had a persistent purulent discharge from behind his ears for six months.

28th October. Signs of illness. Weak pulse; great malaise; nausea; abdominal colic; thirst and sneezing; bowels moving freely which relieved his feelings of illness and pain; cough; sallow complexion.

29th October. 2 or 3 stools during the night, then several more next morning. No temperature throughout the day, no malaise, no colic, so the suspicion of kidney trouble arose because of his foul breath. I prescribed mercury water instead of tea.

Cucumber seed 1 oz; Peeled almonds 10; make up an emulsion with oat water and add to it: Sal Prunella 1½ scruples; Weak cinnamon water 1 oz; Balsamic syrup 1 oz. Take the mixture every 2 hours. Use mercurial water instead of tea.

30th October. Lethargic and sleepy.

Powdered rhubarb root 10 gr; Black mechoacan root 7 gr; Salt of wormwood 1gr; Weak cinnamon water 6 scruples; Solution of rose syrup 2 scruples. Make a potion tomorrow and take it first thing in the morning.

31 October. He took a whole dose of purgative, which made him ill all day. He vomited and produced three stools. In the evening he had a regular, strong pulse. Quite lively, without any pain or feeling of illness.

Make him abstain from oysters, in which he had, against my instructions, indulged in on the previous 2 or 3 days. Use whey and old Rhenish wine. 2 spoonfuls every day, beginning on the 7th day.

November 1st. Rather a restless night; weak, rapid pulse; moderate heat; whitish tongue.

2nd. No febrile heat; tongue looks normal; good appetite and other signs of wellbeing; about evening he had colicky pain and felt ill for half-an-hour.

3rd, 4th and 5th. On the whole quite well, but on the 5th he lost his appetite and felt sleepy. I therefore prescribed a purgative to be taken next morning.

Repeat the purgative draught.

7th. The purgative produced vomiting and 3 stools. Appetite rather better. Temperature rises daily after lunch, especially after eating oysters. I prescribe a tincture.

7th. Rhubarb root 4 scruples; Elecampane root 1½ scruples; Liquorice root 3 scruples; Cochineal 15 gr. Mix in ½ pt of weak cinnamon water and strain. Take 1 spoonful of this

[39] Son of Peter How, the most successful merchant in Whitehaven at this time. He had commercial interests in tobacco, coal, iron, linen, and fishing in Newfoundland. His local positions included those of magistrate, harbour trustee and later turnpike commissioner. He was declared bankrupt in 1763 for £40,000 to £50,000. The family lived in Duke Street. John, the boy described in the case, is buried in St. Nicholas. His tombstone reads: "John, son of Peter How, Esq., & Ann his wife, died 19 December 1737 age 4 years and 7 months".

every day at 7 and 11. Used this tincture for the first 10 days, with the addition of 11 gr of wormwood, but only 1 spoonful of the prescription daily.

18th. Has taken an evacuant tincture which has resulted in one or two motions a day. Appetite now good; occasional bouts of fever; stabbing pains around the eyes without any external signs of inflammation. Weary and weak, but less so than previously. Copious pus now discharging from behind the ears, as was the case before the onset of the illness. He remained in this condition until December 3rd, affected by no other symptoms except troublesome and almost continual discharges. On December 4th I wrote an account of the case history and my methods of treatment and sent it to Dr. Mead. But because of changeable weather, it seemed to me, he developed slight fever and frequent periods of depression, with a whitish tongue. Mrs. How became impatient; Dr. Smelt was sent for.[40] As to what he wrote and the fatal outcome of the disease, see Dr. Mead's description of the case history which is attached.[41]

October, 1736

31 Mrs. Thomas Gale. This woman was about 40 years old, obese and suffering from multiple complaints. She was first affected by pain in the right ear; this was followed by very severe migraine. This pain lasted 3 or 4 days. Laudanum was applied externally as were leeches, and internally she took pain-killing draughts, but on October 30th, her condition having suddenly deteriorated, I was sent for as an emergency.

30th. Pulse rather weak and faster than normal; tongue becoming whitish and dusky, dry and coated; moderate heat; severe thirst; lethargic and very drowsy so that she could hardly be bothered to speak; all sensation of pain was lost; bowels constipated.

N.B. Blood had already been taken from the jugular vein and an enema given. She had had a menstrual period with only scanty loss about the beginning of the illness.

Drank freely of the potion given. Shaved the head and applied a blister.
Black wax water 6 oz; Water of damask rose 1½ oz; Sal Prunella 2 scruples; Elderflower 1½ oz: Make a decoction and take 2 spoonfuls every 2 hours.

31st. In the morning the pulse was stronger; sensation completely restored; terrible strangury, continually trying to pass urine producing only a few drops of blood-stained urine; no headache.

At midday the strangury was really torturing her so I prescribed a mixture to be taken, 1 pt hourly. She drank copiously of barley water and syrup of marshmallow. In the evening, pain from the strangury less; pulse stronger; 1 stool as a result of the enema.

Take the blister from the head and apply a plaster. Husked oats 1 oz; Cream of tartar 3 scruples. Boil until cream of tartar is dissolved in spring water to make up 32 fl. oz. Next, with cucumber seed 1 oz; White poppy seed 3 scruples; 15 drops of almond oil; 5 drops bitter almonds; Hollyhock syrup 2½ oz.
Drink the emulsion freely.
Venetian soap 2 scruples; Camphire 15 gr; Yolk of egg; to this solution add Black wax water 4 oz; Syrup of marshmallow 6 scruples. Inject the enema morning and night.

[40] The story suggests chronic otitis media following measles, culminating in acute bilateral mastoiditis. Brownrigg did not supervise the terminal stage of the disease.

[41] This letter is not in the Casebook.

November 1st. Awake through the night; bowels moved twice; great languor and weakness; pulse regular and of poor volume; pains quite gone. Coughing up thick, dark, mucous material; bad taste in mouth; great fear of death.

November 2nd, 3rd and 4th. Strength grew each day from drinking ½ pt. of moderately strong ale. She lost her voice and was as if drunk and her brain was disturbed for 24 hours. Haemorrhoidal swelling. She did recover, but only by slow stages, for although all her symptoms cleared up, and she had not lost a lot of weight as a result of her illness, nevertheless a great feeling of weakness remained for along time afterwards.

October, 1737

32 Mrs Bouch.[42] This woman who had been married for 3 years but had never been pregnant, was liable to emotional upsets; her monthly periods were very scanty. While she was travelling on the Dublin ferry she became ill with nausea, vomiting, headache and other symptoms of epidemic fever of this type, and in Dublin she was treated for the illness known as nervous fever. On returning home she was seen by me a month after the illness had started.

October 31st. Pulse steady but slow, bowels constipated, tongue dry and coated; but the poor woman was mostly troubled by a sharp pain in the epigastric region which came on every night after her first spell of sleep, and persisted until morning, with troublesome thirst and often with palpitations of the heart, weariness and malaise.

> Rub the epigastric region with linen cloth every day morning and late. Diet for easily digestible foods. Pill Ruffi 1 scruple; Asafoetida 1 scruple; Sal Prunella 1 scruple; enough Peruvian balsam to make up 40 pills. Take 3 morning and late every day. Supplement with 3 pts of this julep:
> Black wax water 1 scruple; Pennyroyal water 1 scruple; Bryony water 6 scruples; Peony water 6 scruples; Tincture of saffron 1½ scruples; Castor oil 1½ scruples; Spirit of lavender 1½ scruples; Syrup of plantain lily 5 scruples. Make the julep.

November 11th. She has taken all the tablets for 3 or 4 days. The pain went away but then returned, then it cleared up and then troubled the poor woman again in turns. I prescribed pills and an electuarium.

> Repeat the pills, laying aside the Sal Prunella and putting cream of tartar in its place and add about ½ scruple of powdered castor. About 15 drops of juniper oil and nut oil. Make the mix and take 4 every night.
> Powdered myrrh 6 scruples; Guaiacum gum 3 scruples; Cream of tartar 2 scruples; Extract of wormwood root 2 oz; Extract and flavour of orange 1 oz; Andromachus treacle 2 scruples; Syrup of plantain lily 2 scruples. Make up the electuary and take it 3 times a day.

November 18th. Her period began but the flow was scanty; but thereafter the pain in her abdomen and the sweating went away.

[42] Martha, wife of John Bouch. Both are buried in St. James's church: 1778, John, aged 88; 1783, Martha, aged 84.

October, 1737

33 Mrs. Drewitt. Puerperal fever. This lady was about 30 years old, of delicate physique and much given to anxious ailments throughout the whole pregnancy and particularly towards term. She had been troubled by vomiting and sickness almost every day, so that her strength was much weakened. She had an uneventful delivery and the lochia were somewhat bulky. At the end of the 3rd week the baby died; as a result, and because of her domestic worries she had serious emotional problems; sickness, heavy precordial pain, almost continuous wakefulness from the time of the birth, constipated bowels, headache and cough, just as in infectious epidemic fever which was common everywhere at the time. Now for a week her bowel symptoms failed to improve but on 29th October she passed many stools, accompanied by colicky pain. This was the beginning of the 4th post-natal week.

October 30th. Signs of illness: Morning, great prostration because of the diarrhoea, pulse steady but very weak, coma, wakefulness, crushing pericardiac pain, headache pain, hence almost perpetual insomnia, with a thousand anxious thoughts; great fear of death; then swollen haemorrhoids, which had bothered her since delivery, disappeared. The diarrhoea settled down; then she had copious sweats and cold shivers by turns, with special sickness after eating or drinking.

Weak cinnamon water 3 oz; Pennyroyal water 3 oz; Bryony water 1½ oz; Tincture of castor 1½ scruples; Saffron 1½ scruples; Syrup of plantain lily 5 scruples. Make up a julep and take 2 pts every half hour. Diet should be easily digestible food with juice taken wisely and freely, but a little at a time, with a few spoonfuls of Canary wine.

October 31st. Moderate bowel movements, sweats and shivers, feeling ill after meals or sleeping.

Repeat the julep.

November 1st. Great fear of death; weariness but pulse stronger and pain somewhat better.

Andromachus treacle 6 scruples; Venetian turpentine 3 scruples; Mace oil 1 scruple. Make a plaster and apply to the stomach region. Warm the feet and ankles with hot water before lying down.

November 2nd. Sweats, gooseflesh and cold shivers, especially after sleep, ill after food, great mental anxiety because of the fear of death and her domestic problems.

November 3rd, 4th and 5th. Strength has returned, but still some abdominal pain at times. Troubled by wind, sickness and weakness but slept better during the night. Once her strength had returned, all her symptoms completely disappeared.[43]

Gum ammoniac 2 scruples: dissolve in 4 oz pennyroyal water and 4 oz black wax water. Castor oil 2 scruples. Take one spoonful every 2 hours on the 5th day.

[43] The only woman with puerperal fever who survived.

November, 1737

34 Mr. Edward Williamson of Parton.[44] A ship's captain, robust, 34 years old. He had suffered first from the bloody flux, and then from diarrhoea for a whole year, then these illnesses cleared up towards the end of last August. Two weeks later, while he was delayed in Dublin, he suddenly started with his present illness there, and after returning home he took all kinds of remedies, to wit, emetics, bitter infusions, volatile drops and decoctions made from Peruvian bark, and venesections.

For his diet he took a little drink of white wine twice or at least 3 times a day.

November 4th. Signs of illness: pulse and respiration normal, bowels rather loose, persistent mild headache, very little appetite, frequent continuous belching for a long time, crushing pain near the scrobiculum which occasionally became worse with a burning sensation not unlike heartburn. This was followed by vertigo with great bodily and mental weakness, slight thirst, tongue suddenly became white and coated. Abdominal pain relieved now and again by spasms of passing wind; great fear of death brought about on the flimsiest pretext. Borborygmi.

Rub the epigastric region with a cloth. Pill Ruffus 2 scruples; Asafoetida 2 scruples; Powdered rhubarb root 2 scruples; Zinc tartar 2 scruples; Peruvian balsam. Make up 12 pills and take a single dose 4 times every morning at 7 and every evening at 8.

November 8th. As a result of taking the pills his bowels became looser and he passed 5 or 6 motions in one day. Very slight headache, occasional vertigo. I ordered an electuary and an infusion.

Electuary for the stomach with myrrh, cream of tartar, etc. Make an infusion with bitter roots and stimulating spices.

About November 16th. Free from all symptoms for 3 or 4 days, then he had an attack of cold shivers, his tongue became white and coated and he began to pass wind up and down. He suddenly developed vertigo and could not see, and yet in a moment he was quite well again. He had great fear of choking from a lump which kept rising in his throat. His bowels were moving regularly.

[Marginal note added later.]

When pain in the head, brain and neck affects a woman and dizziness is seen to affect the eyes, one is afraid she might be depressed, and it is said that black urine and similar uterine discharge can mean anxiety and low spirits. Black bile is in the womb! Hip[pocrates] p.66.[45]

[44] Parton was a small village with a harbour to the north of Whitehaven. Rival coal owners tried to develop this at the expense of the growth of Whitehaven's trade, and several ships' captains had their houses there. Sir James Lowther and the weather prevented Parton's growth, the one through litigation, the other by a series of destructive storms on the exposed coast.

[45] Hippocrates, ed. A. Foesius, *Opera*, Frankfurt, Heirs of A. Wechel, 1595, p. 213. The quotation can be found in *Oeuvres complètes d'Hippocrate*, ed. É Littré, 10 vols, Amsterdam, Adolf M. Hakkert, 1973–89 (hereafter, Littré), vol. 8, *Des maladies des femmes*, bk 2, no. 182, p. 364.

November, 1737

35 Mr. Bodle, a ship's captain in his fifties, robust, partial to spirituous liquors, and suffering greatly from a cough practically every year. At the time when he embarked on his ship on his return from Dublin he was suffering from violent sickness and headache, with rigors and cold sweats in between. After arriving at the Isle of Man, he took emetics there and his sickness settled down, but he was indeed greatly troubled by breathlessness and cough and every day he coughed up large quantities of foul, purulent material, mostly of a dark colour. Three weeks after the start of his illness he returned home.

November 6th. Pulse strong, full but intermittently irregular, breathless with wheezing, cough associated with the copious production of thick mucus, mostly clear, chest pain especially on coughing, bowels loose, tongue coated with filthy exudate and of a livid colour.

> Tolutan Balsam 1 scruple; Native turpentine 2 scruples; Yolk of egg 3 scruples. Pound these well together for a long while and add: Powdered myrrh 6 scruples; Liquorice extract 6 scruples; Pure thick honey 2½ oz. Carefully boil together to reduce to an electuary. Take the above, about the quantity of a nutmeg, every 3 hours with 3 pts of this apozem: Pectoral decoction from the *Edinburgh Pharmacopoeia* 32 oz; Acid oxymel of squills 1 oz. Indulge in horse riding.

December 19th. Now he is fit again and fully back to his condition as he was before his illness. He gradually deteriorated at intervals to a state of chronic troublesome cough with frequent paroxysms, especially at those times when he over-indulged himself in drink made from fermented cereals or the liquor called "punch", so favoured by sailors. His pulse is naturally intermittent.

> Extract of liquorice ½ oz; Myrrh ½ oz; Olibanum ½ oz; Gum sagapenum 3 scruples; Saffron 2 scruples; Castor oil 2 scruples; Peruvian balsam ½ scruple; Turpentine. Make up into pills and use 3 medium-sized pills morning and evening, especially if the cough is troublesome.

November, 1737

36 Mr. Richardson, engineer,[46] a man of good physique, strong and agile, aged 40. Now he had suffered from a fever for a week, being better in the mornings. His head ached severely, his breathing was laboured, and he almost constantly lay awake, his sleep was much disturbed, he had pain in his chest, bowels satisfactory, nausea and vomiting. Blood taken when he was first seen was inflamed and his skin dry.

> His diet should be lighter.

[46] George Richardson was the engineer responsible for the Newcomen engines at Whitehaven which Sir James had installed to aid drainage of the lower levels of his coal pits. By 1737 he was involved with the engine set up at Saltom Pit, the first under-sea coalmine in England. He tried to interest his employers and others in the versatility of the engines, and wrote a paper about the possibility of using them to raise coal from the depths instead of by horse gins. He was killed in a mine explosion on 30th November 1738 and buried in St. Nicholas church.

November 7th. Today his headache is worse and he still has chest pains, wakefulness, a steady pulse, his body and head in particular pour with sweat all day. Urine turbid with a lot of sediment which is whitish and scurfy. Breathing fairly easy.

Shave head and apply a blister.
Fennel root 2 oz; Parsley root 2 oz; Liquorice root 1 ½ oz; Pounded currants 2 oz; Cream of tartar 1 scruple; Nitre 3 scruples. Boil for ½ an hour in spring water to make up 32 oz. Strain. Take 3 cupfuls every 2 hours.

November 8th. Last night was much quieter than before. First thing in the morning he had diarrhoea, extremely profuse sweating, weak pulse, no headache, chest pain fairly slight, tongue dusky in the middle with whitish stringy exudates. Pulse stronger in the evening.

November 9th. Disturbed night, hot with fever, tossing around and delirium. He slept this morning. Skin moist and hot, pulse normal, cough with slight chest pain, lethargy of spirit and body, tongue furred, mouth full of dirty exudate.

November 10th. Disturbed night, hard pulse otherwise normal, but is hot with fever and his breathing rapid and laboured. In the afternoon his pulse was hard and intermittently irregular every 20 or 30 beats, bowels rather constipated, insatiable desire for cold drinks so I prescribed this mixture, for which the patient was most grateful. Humours in the mouth rather thick.

Hyssop water 4 oz; Pennyroyal water 4 oz; Wax water 4 oz; Vitriolated tartar 1 scruple; Sal Prunella 3 scruples; Tamarind syrup 2 oz; Rob. of elderflower 1 oz. Make a mixture and take one spoonful every hour.

November 11th. Wakeful and restless all night. Had a light sleep in the morning and on waking was quietly confused, slight fever, skin moist, pulse regular and almost normal, but a little hard.

Repeat the prescribed mixture.

November 12th. Pulse weak and empty, skin moist and sticky. Last night much quieter than preceding ones, light naps without sleep or delirium, slight fever. Vomiting and illness in the evening.

November 13th. Restless night without sleep, headache with the pain being mainly occipital, vomited back his medicine, mouth sticky, thick perspiration. During the morning the pains settled down, pulse remained weak and irregular, laboured breathing, skin sticky, feverish. In the afternoon, copious thick perspiration, pulse regular, urine at first full of reddish streaks and afterwards a considerable whitish deposit and it remained turbid.

November 14th and the next few days. Still copious, viscous, offensive sweat for 2 days. This then improved his symptoms. His appetite improved and his strength gradually returned.

Drank copiously of Bristol water.

October 31st, 1737

37 Mr. Grindale's daughter, aged 5 years. She was seized by a fever. Pulse was as strong as possible, rapid and hard, breathing rapid and laboured, dry skin, tongue dusky and coated with white exudate. She complained sometimes of pain now in her head, now in her side, now her throat, moreover she was very restless and wanted to lie in a single bed, nor could she bear to be touched. She refused all foods and medicines, and by way of drinks she took ale and almond emulsion, and these only in very small doses, about the fourth day of her illness. A softening enema was injected and a vermifuge plaster was applied to the epigastric area. On the 6th day she was comatose and I prescribed the plaster described opposite [see below] to be applied to the soles of her feet for up to 4 days. Her bowels remained constipated until the 9th, then she was affected by abdominal colic and after 4 or 5 motions the fever cleared up beyond the hope of her friends.

> Plaster the head with a strained gum mixture made without spurge 4 parts.
> A blistering plaster—part 1.
> Make a plaster to apply to the feet.

November 1st, 1737

38 Mr. Poe's son, a boy aged 7½, of good condition. This boy had suffered from a fever of the inflammatory kind for a week. He had been bled three times and the blood obtained was inflamed and turbid. His present symptoms are the same as before.

> Before I was called in, blood had been drawn 3 times, enemas had been administered, and linctus and other pectoral medicines had been tried.

Pulse hard, full and strong with the artery rather stiff and slowly dilating and contracting. Breathing rapid and irregular and laboured even after great effort. He produced a sort of sobbing noise when breathing out, with a great fear of suffocation. He had a most troublesome little cough, occasional sickness, headache and pain in the side which was really sharp. When the pain occasioned upset, his throat was extremely sore, so that he could hardly breathe. He was very restless at night and was quiet but delirious on waking. Scarcely any thirst, but skin dry. I took care to bleed him again twice. The blood remained somewhat inflamed, nor did his pain settle, only decrease. On about November 6th his bowels then moved twice with great relief and gradually he recovered following this.

> I prescribed 2 more bleedings and a pectoral apozem against fever. Softening enemas and a light diet.

October, 1737

39 Infant of Mr. Dent,[47] 5 months old, of good bodily condition and previously free from all disease. The mother, who was breast-feeding the child, was an obese young woman of relaxed fibre and much more given to emotional disturbances. For a week she had been suffering from abdominal pain and wind and for this she had been drinking a purgative

[47] John, son of George Dent, an officer (probably of Customs). The child died in 1741.

potion made from senna, manna and similar soothing ingredients. The baby had the same disease as his mother and having been given purgatives he moved his bowels more often than his mother.

8th October (evening). Next day, that is to say October 8th, the child was seized with convulsions and his little body was stiff as a stone and he passed wind both up and down. His bowels have moved 4 or 5 times today—stools green at times.

> Mr. Sanderson injected a relaxing enema and a mixture composed of pulverised shells, clear water, aniseed oil and diacord syrup. I should recommend use of these. I also prescribed 1 scruple of diacord syrup to be taken as soon as possible and a treacle plaster applied to the epigastric region.

October 9th. Very disturbed night, and he had frequent epileptic attacks accompanied by crying. There were 2 yellow motions, no fever. I prescribed a powder and as a result he passed 6 or more motions and his pain settled. In the afternoon I prescribed a mixture which he took readily.

> 7 grains of rhubarb; 1 grain of wormwood; 4 grains of red coral. Take by appropriate means.

After taking the mixture I ordered and the other nutritious foods I had recommended, the baby appeared to be quite well for a whole week, but then the abdominal convulsions returned once more, together with the other symptoms.

> Venetian soap 2 scruples; Aniseed oil 3 drops; Egg yolk 1 ½ scruples; Pound together well and mix in Mint water 2½ oz and Syrup of marshmallow 1 oz. Take one spoonful every hour.

On examining the motions I found them to be yellow and mixed with clotted white specks of milk. By means of rhubarb and the other remedies I have described the baby was completely restored to his former health.

> Repeat powders with rhubarb. Inject the following enema as soon as possible:
> Spring water 2 oz; Cow's milk 2 oz; Almond oil ½ oz; Wormwood 6 grains. Reduce to a watery liquid and inject. Suckling to be replaced by bread, meat and other warming things.

November 14th, 1737

40 Mrs. Barrow,[48] a widow about 40 years old of good constitution and full of sap, taking only watery drinks and abstaining from fermented liquors whence she had a weakness of the stomach. A cough had affected her since childhood with thick sputum and frequent vomiting. Her periods were always regular.

Signs of illness: In the morning of 14th she complained of a headache. For breakfast she drank 2 cups of tea. About twelve midday she suddenly fell to the ground completely paralysed and unconscious. Her bladder sphincter relaxed and she was incontinent of

[48] Formerly Elizabeth Stockdale, she was married to Robert Barrow, a mariner, in St. Nicholas church on 30 September 1718.

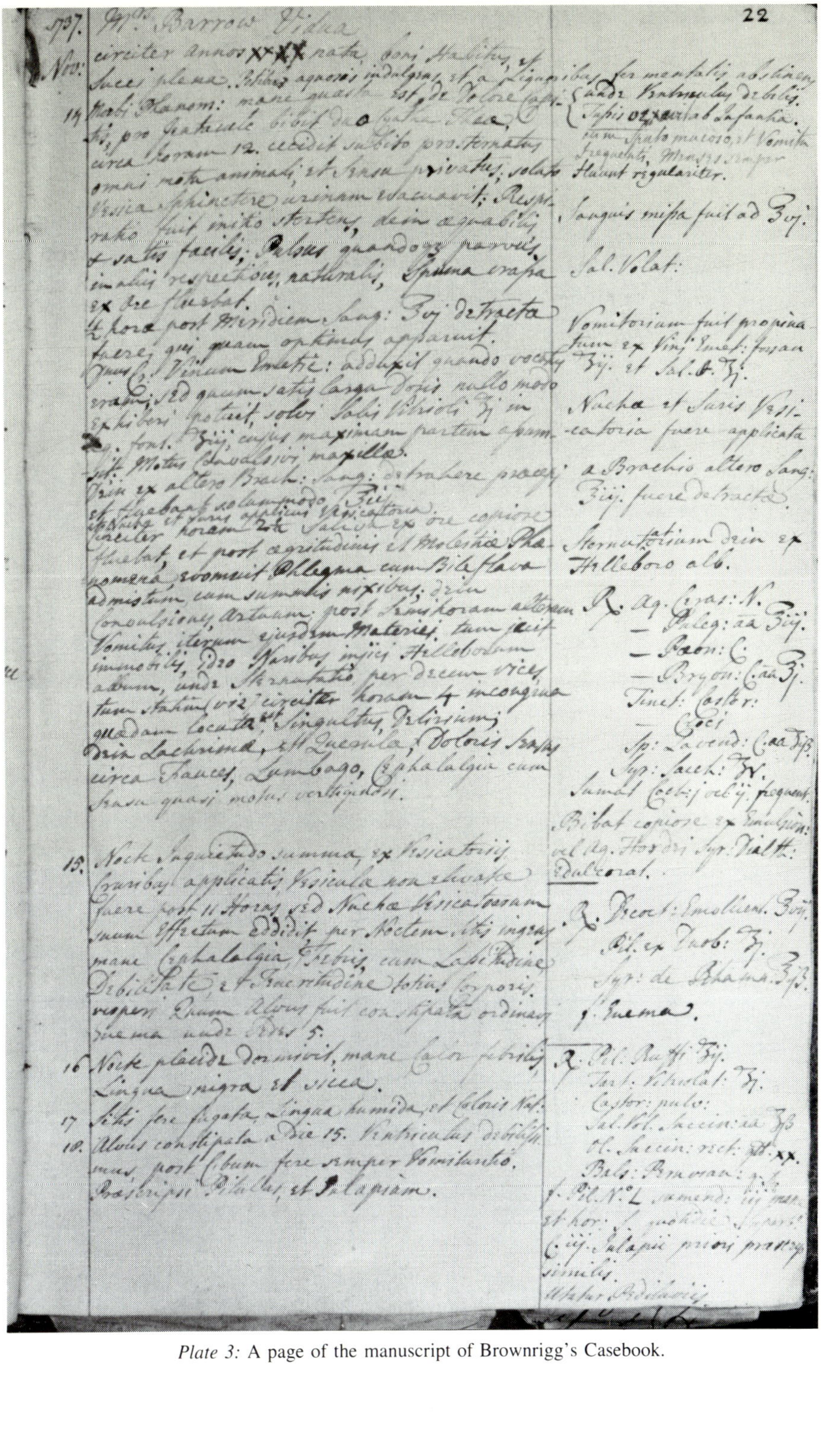

Plate 3: A page of the manuscript of Brownrigg's Casebook.

urine. Breathing stertorous at first, later more regular and fairly easy, pulse small at times but otherwise normal, thick froth poured from her mouth. At half past twelve 6 oz of blood were drawn and this appeared in good condition.

> Blood let to the quantity of 6 oz. Sal Volatile. Made a vomiting drink from emetic wine (perhaps 2 oz) and 1 oz of salt.

When I was called, Mr. Creighton had attempted to give her a wine emetic, but as she was quite unable to take a sufficiently large dose, I dissolved Vitriol salt in 3 oz spring water and she swallowed most of this. Her jaws were shaking convulsively and I now advised blood to be taken from the other arm, about 3 oz. Vesicatories were applied to the back of the neck and calves of the legs.

> Blistering ointments were applied to the neck and calves of the legs. 3 oz of blood were extracted from the other arm.

About half past two copious saliva poured from her mouth and after this episode came some signs of malaise and trouble. She vomited phlegm mixed with yellow bile after great efforts, then came convulsions of the limbs. Half an hour later she vomited the same material again. Then she lay quite still, so I instilled white hellebore into her nostrils, which made her sneeze ten times.

> She was made to sneeze with white hellebore.

Then suddenly about four o'clock she spoke a few incoherent words with some sobbing and delirium. After this she wept and complained of a painful sensation in her throat, lumbago and a headache with a feeling of dizziness.

> Barley water 3 oz; Pennyroyal water 3 oz; Peony water 3 oz; Bryony water 3 oz; Tincture of castor; Tincture of saffron; Lavender spirit 1 ½ scruples; Sugar syrup 5 scruples. Take 1 or 2 spoonfuls. Drink copiously from the emulsion or barley water, sweetened with syrup of marshmallow.

November 15th. A very restless night. More vesicatories were applied to her legs. No blisters were raised after eleven hours, but there was a blister from the vesicatory on the back of the neck. She was very thirsty during the night. In the morning headache, fever, weariness, and weakness with the tenderness of her whole body. In the evening, she was constipated, I ordered an enema. Result 5 stools.

> Emollient decoction 7 oz; Double pill 1 scruple; Buckthorn syrup 1 ½ oz. Make an enema.

November 16th. Slept peacefully all night. In the morning fever, and tongue blackish and dry.

November 17th. Thirst almost gone. Tongue moist and normal colour.

November 18th. Bowels constipated since the 15th. Very weak stomach with vomiting after every meal. I prescribed pills and a julep.

Pill Ruffi 2 scruples; Vitriolated tartar 1 scruple; Ground sugar ½ scruple; Amber sal volatile ½ scruple; Amber oil 20 drops in the rectum. Enough Peruvian bark to make 50 pills. Take 3 in the morning and at 5 each day. Take 3 pts of the julep like that previously described. Footbaths are to be used.

November, 1737

41 Mrs. Carlisle Spedding,[49] an obese woman of 40, given to mental trouble, and leucophlegmatic. Several years ago she had jaundice which was serious and affected her for a long time afterwards, then she had two further, but less serious, episodes of the same illness. She had been troubled by discomfort in the region of the stomach with frequent vomiting of yellow bile in the mornings, and discomfort increases as the vomit grows less. Now for six months she has been troubled by frequent nosebleeds. When the bleeding stops her nose becomes blocked up and she feels as if she has a head cold, and troubled by catarrh.

N.B. She takes spirituous liquors from time to time.

Indications: To strengthen the fibres of the stomach and the whole body. To improve the necessary concoctions and excretions. To draw off and eliminate the excess humours. To pay attention to the formation of bile so as to remove, or at least guard against, obstructions of the liver.

November 16th. So as to achieve these aims I have ordered these pills:

Rhubarb root as prescribed. Rabbit's blood as prescribed. Myrrh 2 scruples; Pure aloe juice 2 scruples; Amber sal volatile ½ scruple; Amber oil 20 drops by rectum; Balsam of copaiba, enough to make a mass of hard consistency and enough to make 100 pills. Take 4 of these every morning and night.

November 20th, 1737

42 Miss Robinson of Egremond.[50] A girl of 15 who for 8 years had been tormented by ischuria and terrible pain in the lower part of the abdomen. But since she only suffered at intervals and sometimes remained well for 6 months at a time, free from all pain; as she did not show any signs of nephritis, nor passed any stones, Dr. Askew thought that her illness was due to acid urine and he prescribed an electuary and astringent warm wash which are here described:

Dr. Askew's electuary was composed of: Pearl; Crabs eyes; Red coral; Guaiacum gum; Sal martis; Andromachus treacle and other conserves. The warming wash was with a decoction of oak bark and other restringents applied to the hypogastrium.

On several occasions he thought her symptoms were relieved by these substances. To these Dr. Askew added treatment of his own. Dr. Senhouse prescribed only well-fermented strong ale and whey. And now that her pains had returned and Spring had passed she felt no relief from treatment with her usual remedies, indeed the pain became

[49] Sarah, wife of Carlisle Spedding, the mining engineer employed by Sir James Lowther (see Case No. 57). She was described by her contemporaries as a shrewish woman, but her ill-health may have accounted for this, coupled with the constant anxiety she must have felt for her husband, carrying out a most dangerous employment and often debilitated as a result of going into unsafe mine workings.

[50] Egremont, a town five miles south of Whitehaven.

much worse. She developed slight fever and the illness persisted so that in addition I treated her with gum arabic, decoction of mallow, clysters and other strong remedies.

Signs of illness: Emaciation and slight slow fever. She had unremitting supra-pubic pain, especially on the left side. At night this pain was greatly increased and she felt hot and thirsty. She had very severe pain along with convulsive movements on passing urine, which she often passed with some difficulty and only a few drops at a time. During the night her urine trickled continually and imperceptibly from her. Tenesmus on passing urine. Formerly the urine had been stringy but clear, but now it was thick and with a white sediment and heavily laden with mucus. Sometimes it was mixed with a purulent material. Recently, grains like sand have been observed being passed with urine.

So as to prevent abrasions, irritation and inflammation of the bladder and to reduce the violent contractions, I prescribed an electuary and I also prescribed laudanum in liquid and powder form and as a result her pain settled slightly.

> Myrrh 2 scruples; Gum mastic 2 scruples; Type of diatrag. to make up 3 scruples;[51] Pure manna 6 scruples; Liquorice extract 3 scruples; Extract of pulp of fresh senna 2 oz; Marshmallow syrup. By mixing exactly, make the electuary. Take an amount the size of a nutmeg 3 times daily an hour before breakfast, luncheon or dinner. Drink the above dose with whey.
> Type of diatrag. 1 scruple; Crabs eyes 1 scruple; Gum arabic ½ scruple. Crush together and take one dose at dawn and night with milk.

She was then affected by the most terrible torments, severe wasting and slow fever. At length, about the beginning of June, she died.

The end of October, 1737

43 Miss Catharine Copeland, a girl aged 10. Her father suffered from phthisis at the time her mother became pregnant. The girl was beautiful but delicate and in the preceding year or two suffered from hectic fever. About the month of October, however, she began to suffer from a similar fever, losing her appetite, with a fast, weak pulse and dry skin. The fever was always worse towards evening with sciatic pains and nightly sweatings. She was prostrated by this illness until the beginning of January by which time I had been called in and prescribed an electuary.

> Best myrrh 1½ scruples; Gum mastic 1½ scruples; Powdered crabs eyes 3 scruples; Wormwood conserve 1 oz; Syrup of Tunica. Make an electuary. Take an amount the size of a small nutmeg every morning. For a drink: Cow's milk and Bristol water. Drink Bristol water with an equal amount of cow's milk for her everyday drink.

Meanwhile the pain in her hips and thighs disappeared, but her upper and lower legs were paralysed so that she was unable to walk or move her toes. However, these parts still retained heat and slight feeling. At the end of January her appetite improved, the febrile exudations less often recurred and the sweats vanished. Strength and movement were unexpectedly restored to her limbs and so suddenly that on feet which were lame in the

[51] Diatrag—we have not been able to trace this substance.

morning she was able to stand and walk at noon as well and firmly as she had done before. From then on she took an infusion of yellow amaranth and in a short time she put on weight and recovered all her strength.

Infusion of yellow amaranthus 12 oz; Spirit of lavender 1 scruple; Astringent of Helvia 2 oz; Wormwood water 2 oz.

October, 1737

44 Mrs. Gregg of Cockermouth,[52] a woman of 53, of obese habit, affected by dropsy for 10 years and having had no monthly flow for 3 years. She indulged herself in thick, fatty foods and too many vinous liquors. She had an excess of serous fluid as is clear from a lump which appeared on her leg. She was also troubled by pain in her kidneys caused by gravel.

October 15th. Seven days had elapsed since she was beset by fever, accompanied by thirst and a cough with no sputum but difficulty in breathing. Her stools were frequent and watery and streaked with blood, like water in which meat is washed, a copious flow, they were neither slimy nor offensive and were not accompanied by severe colic. Her stools between times were firm and free from blood. A month before this, after riding she had passed these same bloody stools but with a small flow, 4 or 5 times before that. The first evacuation of this sort happened 5 years ago. The fever has ended, but the remainder of her symptoms persist, violently tortured by thirst and with growing pain in her back from shoulders to hips but spreading all over her body. She was very restless and sleepless. Her tongue is scurfy, dry, whitish, foul. Before I was called she was given restringents and strengthened opiates. At night I prescribed for her a better draught than she had received.

Hyssop water 1 oz; Sweet almond oil ½ oz; Liquid laudanum 14 drops; Hartshorn spirit 15 drops; Balsamic syrup 1 scruple. Take the draught as prescribed.

October 16th. On the following morning I made a pill with which her stomach was loosened 5 times without cramps, or malaise, nor were any serous humours seen. At bedtime I prescribed the draught to be repeated.

Powdered rhubarb ½ oz; Sal Prunella 10 gr; Cinnamon oil ½ drop; Rose syrup. Make up the pill. Repeat the prescribed draught.

October 18th. She took the purgative bolus again, with the addition of 5 gr rhubarb, with which she had 5 stools but she was unwilling to take the paregoric. This should help her diet: a little green tea with rice milk, canary whey or with beestings; very weak coffee and by way of an ordinary drink, Bristol water with one part in four of red wine. For lunch, very tender young meat with toast and stewed fruit. She is not to take any fish, firm meat or fatty foods. The parts affected by pain in the abdomen should be rubbed with Welsh cloth for ½ hr daily.

October 20th. Since with this treatment all her symptoms were somewhat improved and the serous discharge virtually ceased, I prescribed a decoction.

[52] Cockermouth is a town about 15 miles north-east of Whitehaven.

Fresh fennel root 2 oz; Burberry root 1½ oz; Sorrel root 1½ oz; Liquorice root 1 oz; Confection of currants 2 oz; Sal Prunella 3 scruples. Boil in spring water. Make up to 2 pts. Strain until clear and take 4 spoonfuls every 3 hours daily.

December 10th, 1737. She rapidly recovered with this treatment. She was suffering from a cough and cold in the head, so was complaining of pains in her back. First she had one or two nosebleeds and then she passed a large quantity of serous blood from the bowel. She took two of the pills I prescribed and again recovered.

[Later insert in the margin for prescriptions.]

Disquisition upon the nature of her illness: When the sick woman swelled with pus and serous fluid and her sweating was obstructed (as the cough shows) many serous humours are squashed together, which are driven out through the relaxed vessels in the small intestines as if by a spasm. Another part of these flows into the lungs via the trachea, stimulates the nerves, and agitates the cough. These veins running by the lungs are blocked of humours, which cause difficulty in breathing. Lumbago seems to arise either by the obstruction or irritation of the nerves, but this always was seen to begin before an evacuation. This, therefore, was seen to be the primary effect of the illness and it would be removed when the cause of the illness was treated. The following points have a bearing on the case. To evacuate the offending humours, to check their excessive stickiness, and to make them freely flow through the vessels. Then to strengthen the vessels and prevent a fresh massing of these humours.

November, 1737

45 Mr. Samuel Thompson, Mr. Gale's[53] servant, a temperate man of about 60 and something of an invalid. For many years he had suffered from a phlegmy cough and wheezing. Recently he has been troubled by vertigo and headaches often, and in the last 6 months he has had two similar attacks of slight apoplexy with convulsions.

November 21st. He complained of headache all day; at night he had hardly got into bed before a sudden stroke rendered him unconscious and paralysed. I was a witness to this episode.

I found his pulse normal, breathing stertorous and his jaws clamped tightly together. His eyes were fixed, he was yawning frequently and his eyes and limbs were jerking spasmodically from time to time. His whole body was bathed in perspiration. He vomited once before I could approach him, and produced thick, frothy phlegm from his mouth.

Extracted 8 oz blood from an arm vein, then used 1 scruple of salt of vitriol dissolved in ½ oz of spring water. With great effort he brought up thick viscous black phlegm, nearly always with his teeth clenched tightly together.
A large blister was applied to the back of his neck. He also swallowed volatile drops in water.

No remedies had any effect and five hours later he died from the stroke.

[53] The Gales were a prominent merchant family.

About October 15th, 1737

46 Mrs. Berbeck,[54] a woman of about 60, a regular drinker, of good temperament and healthy. About the middle of October she was first struck down by a hemiplegia, then with a brief but severe stroke. Six hours after this first attack I was called in. I could not relieve her symptoms with venesection or blistering or inhalations, although her pulse was quite strong, full and regular. She died about 8 o'clock from the stroke.

November 1st, 1737

47 Mrs. Richardson, a widow aged 56. She was already suffering from a cough and epidemic inflammatory fever, with lassitude and weakness when she suddenly fell, paralysed and unconscious. She vomited and was incontinent of a large quantity of urine and then, after a short interval of time, became quite well again, except that for a few days she was troubled by stomach pains.[55]

November 24th, 1737

48 Mr. Dan[iel], Pee's servant. A robust 21-year-old sailor who had been suffering from diarrhoea while sailing from Virginia. As soon as he reached port about a week ago he was attacked by a fever which continued until the 20th. Blood was taken. His fever became worse today and he was affected by pleuritic pain. The venesection was repeated and emulsions, antiseptic powders and a linctus were prescribed.

> Note: He must drink copious diluting fluids. Footbath at 10 a.m. He must continue to take the medicines that are already helping him. His head to be shaved.

Signs of illness: Pulse rapid, small and regular; skin hot and dry; laboured breathing, much troubled by a very irritating persistent non-productive cough, headache and a tendency to mental confusion. His pleuritic pain had cleared up but he was suffering from other widespread aches and pains. Blood very inflamed with flakes and leathery strings of clots. Tongue moist and rather whitish, no great thirst. Urine stringy and full of suspended material, bowels somewhat loose.

November 25th. Slept at night. Troubled by an occasional irritating little cough, with headache. Pulse a little stronger, but very rapid. Sleep disturbed by quiet delirium. Bowels loose.

> A decoction for the heart from the *Edinburgh Pharmacopoeia*, 2 pts in quantity. To this add between meals: Pure nitre 3 scruples; Sea holly 3 scruples; Tamarind fruit 1 oz. Take 4 spoonfuls every 2 hrs. At bedtime apply a vesicatory to the head.

November 26th and the next few days. Tongue drier and dusky in colour, headache less, cough now producing copious thin sputum which is gradually becoming thicker. I prescribed a decoction and linctus to be taken every time he had something to drink, or less frequently if circumstances demanded. So his fever gradually cleared up over a period of a

[54] Christian, wife of Thomas Berbeck, an officer of militia. She was buried in Holy Trinity church.

[55] Cases 45–47 are all written on a single page. Brownrigg was obviously connecting them under similar symptoms. Perhaps he was trying to assess why Mrs. Richardson had survived, while the other two died.

week, but the pain in his side remained persistent and his cough lasted much longer after all his other symptoms had disappeared completely.

Decoction for the chest from the *Edinburgh Pharmacopoeia*—2 pts; Pure nitre 3 scruples. Strain and add oxymel of squills 6 scruples. Our linctus fortified with almond oil, opium and rose hip conserve.

1737

49 An apprentice of Mr. Hicks. A young man aged 20, formerly robust and healthy. He suffered an inflammatory fever about the same time and with the same symptoms as the preceding case. He was venesected 3 times at intervals and treated with large quantities of nitrous salts. About the eighth day of the illness he brought up copious amounts of sputum. I prescribed an apozem, etc., and about the 15th day he recovered completely.[56]

December 15th, 1737

50 Mrs. Taylor, a woman aged 40, of frail physique, often subjected to attacks of coughing and asthma which always responded to a draught of laudanum. Four years ago she was delivered of a dead male child, her first, during the eighth month of pregnancy while she was suffering from pleurisy, and she was somewhat weakened by a copious loss of blood. (She is of cachectic temperament and has often suffered from rheumatics, and in the past from wasting ulcers of the legs.) Now she is aware once more of the signs of pregnancy, to wit: her menstrual periods, which formerly occurred regularly, have not appeared for 3 months; for the whole of this time she has suffered from malaise and morning sickness and in addition her breasts are swelling.

About ten weeks from the time she suspected she had conceived, florid blood of normal consistency issued from the vaginal orifice every time she moved her bowels. Blood was let, and she took to drinking red wine mixed with water. As a result her bowels became more constipated and this increased the vaginal loss. Now this symptom has lasted for 3 weeks, her legs are swelling in the evenings, and abdominal colic has occurred at intervals near the pubic area, especially when she moves her bowels, but without any evidence of labour pains. She has also been taking vinegar with a large quantity of mercury which causes nausea and vomiting, especially if she drinks it in the mornings.

Within a week of taking the prescribed medicines all her pains and colic ceased completely and the blood loss was rather less, but when her bowels were more controlled and needed a great effort in defaecating, the blood was flowing. Instead of the pills I prescribed a bolus for 2 nights which produced 3 stools daily and all her symptoms cleared up.

16th December. Took 8 oz of blood from an arm vein.
Rhubarb; Powdered hematite stone 2 scruples; Gum lacca 2 scruples; Oil of cinnamon 8 drops; Peruvian bark, enough to make up 24 pills. Take 3 morning and night every day. Take 3 spoonfuls of this julep with the above.
Milky alexipyretic water 3 oz; Weak cinnamon 3 oz; Strong cinnamon 1½ oz; Damask rose 1 oz; 30 drops of Sydenham's narcotic draught; Pearl 2 scruples; Gum arabic 1

[56] Cases 48 and 49 were written on the same page. Was Brownrigg considering the possibility of Hick's apprentice having been infected by the fever brought from Virginia?

scruple; White sugar 2 scruples. Make into a julep.
Repeat the pills and the julep.
Best powdered rhubarb; Gum mastic ½ scruple; Gum lacca ½ scruple; Syrup of diacord. Make into a bolus to be taken instead of the pills. Her body was rubbed all over.

January 16th. During the last three or four days her cough and wheezing have increased her misery, and a few drops of blood have trickled from her vagina when she has moved her bowels. During all this time she has taken the pills, three of which were to be taken once daily, and she now has had recourse to her sacred sheet anchor, laudanum. Meanwhile pains and colic have sharply troubled the wretched woman, and they can be relieved by laudanum alone. Indeed at this time she has been suffering from considerable depression. I prescribe:

Type of diamb. 1 scruple; Powdered amber 1 scruple; Gum mastic 1½ scruples; Andromachus treacle 2 scruples; Conserve of wormwood 6 scruples; Tunica syrup. Make an electuary. Take every day with 4 spoonfuls of the following: ½ pt of simple, bitter drink. To this add at the time of infusion, Iris root 3 scruples; Elecampane root 3 scruples; Strain and add wormwood water 4 oz; Spirit of lavender 1½ scruples.

See page 45.[57]

1737/8. Mrs. Taylor, from page 26.

The month of January. I prescribed pills with a dose of rhubarb, one dose every day for a week, from which her bowels responded twice in the one day and her flow of blood was entirely checked.

Months of February and March. She frequently suffered from rheumatism in the arms and shoulders, from which she was tormented with misery. In April the pains indeed moderated but gradually there arose a weakness of the whole body, of such a nature of depression of spirits and tiredness that she was scarcely able to speak for several days. Laudanum always soothed her worries and pains and she continually used small doses of it every night. However, around the very beginning of June she delivered a lively robust son at full term. Three or four days after the birth she was afflicted with breathlessness and with a whistling of breath. However, with a short use of laudanum and a mixture of gums it was quietened, and with her lochia flowing away normally, she grew better and vigorous despite expectations to the contrary.

December 21st, 1737, 4th day of illness.

51 Edward Bradford,[58] a sailor who died of epidemic inflammatory fever. A robust man of 32 who suddenly became ill with a fever on 18th December. On 20th, Mr. Smith took 12 oz blood from his arm and prescribed various antiseptic powders. The pain in his chest, which had previously caused the patient the greatest distress, was greatly relieved. The blood was of a leathery colour and rather inflamed, with a large amount of yellowish serum. Pulse now small, but regular and rapid, laboured breathing, quite troublesome

[57] The remainder of her case is described on page 45 of the original Casebook. It has been brought forward here to maintain continuity.

[58] Buried in St. Nicholas church.

cough with vomiting, severe thirst, dry shiny tongue, diarrhoea, chest pain, lancinating head pains especially when coughing, widespread pains and lassitude, urine very turbid without sediment and of a pale, reddish colour.

Drew 7 oz of blood. Shaved head and applied an epispastic.
Cold seeds of house leek 1 oz; White poppy ½ oz; Almond oil No. 20. Mix with barley water, make up to 2 pts of an emulsion. Add to it:
Nitre 3 scruples; Syrup of marshmallow 1 ½ oz; Take 4 spoonfuls of the mixture alternate hours.

Day 5 of illness. Rather a disturbed night, quietly confused. 5 or 6 stools passed. In the morning, pulse rather weak and rapid, severe thirst, all pain improved, cough much less, vomiting and malaise. The last blood taken was watery and pale yellow and with many leathery threads and clots. Skin normal to the touch with no fever.

In the evening. Apply blistering ointment to the legs.

Day 6 of illness. Much worse in every way. Skin fairly hot to the touch, pulse very weak, respirations deep and slow with stertorous wheezing and only possible with great effort, coma, unquenchable thirst, filthy tongue, delirium.

6 o'clock. Plasters on the area of the feet, the same as the head plasters but divided in two and with 3 epispastics.

At 6 o'clock in the evening his pulse increased in volume and grew stronger and he was sticky with perspiration. He died at 9 o'clock.

December, 1737/8

52 Mrs. Wood, a raffler's[59] wife. A woman of about 35, very obese and suffering from an umbilical hernia. For 3 days before the birth of her child she had been ill with a cough and slight fever. She had a perfectly normal delivery and milk was expressed from the breasts. About the fifth day after delivery she had a little fever with a most troublesome unproductive cough. Dr. Wood was consulted and he prescribed a laxative enema, a linctus, and poultices to be applied next day to both legs, and he ordered strengthening boluses with julep to be taken every 5 hours. She took 12 of these. The fever was greatly aggravated by this treatment; she suffered great thirst and said that the whole of her inside was on fire because of these boluses. Her tongue became quite black. After this, when vesicatories had been applied, all the lower parts became paralysed, so that she could only move her arms and her head. In addition, the lochia were red and flowing copiously. Mr. Smith and the midwife gave her emulsions, pain-killing and binding mixtures, but with no relief to the patient and twice they complied with the patient's demands and gave her strong beer.

Boluses from Dr. Wood.
American mulberry 31 gr; Saffron 6 gr; Castor 6 gr; Camphor 2 gr; Confection of Kermes. These made up the bolus.

[59] A raffler was a person who sold china ornaments, usually by hawking them in public houses.

December 28th. On the 14th day after delivery I was asked to see her. As well as all the previous symptoms, her chest and brain were now affected, for her breathing was rapid and stertorous with wheezing, and while awake she was quietly delirious all the time. Her sleep was very disturbed, pulse rapid and weak, today her face is perspiring, deafness, tenderness all over her body. Thin fluid is flowing profusely from vesicatories.

I prescribed a light diet.
Almond oil 2 scruples; Tolutan balsam ½ scruples; Venetian soap 6 gr; Egg yolk 3 scruples; Hyssop water 1 oz; Weak cinnamon water ½ oz; Liquid balsam 2 scruples. Drink 1/6 of this every hour.
Hyssop water 2½ scruples; Weak cinnamon water 2½ scruples; Sal Prunella 1½ scruples; Spirit of sulphur and camphor 20 drops; Oxymel of squills 2 oz; Balsamic syrup 1 oz. Concoct the mixture and take 3 spoonfuls every 3 hours after one drink. Drink freely of the prescribed emulsion.

December 29th. Previous signs of fever somewhat improved, breathing still wheezy but less than before. As the bowels have not moved for 2 days I have prescribed a suppository. This produced a motion. In the evening a very rapid pulse, extremely restless, great thirst, very severe pain in the side which was relieved by warm water and frothy milk. About 2 o'clock in the following morning, she died.

Persist in using the prescription, without soap.
Coltsfoot leaves 1 minim; Maidenhair 1 minim; Root of sea holly 3 scruples; Iris flower 3 scruples; Crushed currants 2 oz. Boil these for half-an-hour in 2 pts of spring water. Add 10 scruples of liquorice at the end and nitre 3 scruples; Honey 3 scruples. Drink 6 spoonfuls frequently.

November, 1737

53 Mr. Key, a ship's captain aged 31, of good constitution and accustomed to hard work and formerly apt to indulge to some extent in drinking. Now for many years he had suffered from cough and dyspnoea which affected him without any known preceding cause. He took various remedies but with no relief. Indeed, during the last episode, Boerhaave prescribed pills made of liquorice extract and myrrh in equal proportions. In the autumn Mr. Harrison ordered a mixture of emetics, Peruvian bark, balsam, Peruvian sulphur, and on the most recent occasion he used liquid tar in quite large amounts, which produced vomiting and diarrhoea.

November 8th. Signs of illness: Weak, rapid pulse, fever, breathlessness, a very troublesome cough affecting him especially at night, with copious white, tenacious frothy sputum consisting mainly of mucus. Tongue dirty and dusky in colour, great thirst, appetite completely absent, colicky diarrhoea and in addition complete weakness of the stomach so that he vomited after the lightest of meals and he had a hoarse and most painful throat.

Nature of the illness: The chylopoietic and haemopoietic organs are not functioning properly, as a result many of the humours are viscous and sluggish. The phlegmatic humours which are not being properly circulated are accumulating in the bloodstream and from thence are expelled, via the somewhat weakened exhaling vessels in the lungs, into the aerating pulmonary vessels. There is as a result a drying-up and thickening of these most fluid parts until the body is in the prone position. These humours go down into the main branches of the bronchial tree and then, after a much prolonged effort has brought about a fit of coughing they are spat out looking like phlegm, viscous, frothy, etc. Bennet has observed that this type of phlegm is of the same nature as the nourishing humours, and that the blood serum clots with heat. In this case the body ceases to be nourished, because of debility of the whole body rather than from damage to any particular organ.

I prescribed various remedies in an attempt to relieve his illness, but to no avail. About the middle of December, without any sign of pain or malaise, he died from suffocation.

Diet should be whey, rice pudding, juice, apples, roasted meat of young animals. The abdomen is to be rubbed with woollen cloth, and exercise on horseback befriending the weather.
Tormentil root ½ scruple; Powdered hartshorn ½ scruple; Coral ½ scruple; Slightly-cooked green rhubarb 6 gr. Take with chicken every morning with milk. Use this and abstain from spicy liquids. Vomiting ceased but he was troubled by diarrhoea just as before.
Gum mastic 2 scruples; Myrrh 2 Scruples; Ammoniac gum 2 scruples; Extract of liquorice 2 scruples; Peruvian bark, enough to make up pills of 5 gr. Take 3 every day.
As the diarrhoea was troublesome, pills of more restringency were prescribed, with the addition of catachu, but there was no relief, and a restringent enema, but no success. However, before he died I made up an electuary and confection with which the diarrhoea was contained a little.

January 1st, 1738

54 Mr. Fausett, a ship's captain, a man in his fifties, employed in the coal trade[60] and, as is the custom among such men, much given to indulging in the drinking of spirits. Towards the end of October he fell ill with a cough and other symptoms which had never troubled him before.

Signs of illness: Slow, small pulse, breathlessness on slightest exertion, very troublesome cough especially at night, with sputum similar to that described in the preceding case, the history of Mr. Key, that is to say frothy, whitish and odourless. Hoarse throat, weakness and prostration, no appetite, bowels regular. In the previous year his brother had died from the same illness, but no other member of his family had suffered from a wasting condition.

N.B. His brother had died from dysentery caught in America, not from phthisis.

Light diet of milk. Rubbing the body morning and evening. Myrrh 1 scruple; Gum mastic 1 scruple; Extract of liquorice 1 scruple; Giant fennel 1 scruple; Castor oil 1 scruple; Saffron 1 scruple; Ammon 1 scruple; Aniseed oil 12 drops; Nutmeg oil 12 drops; Venetian turpentine; Extract of heather 1 scruple. Make 10 pills and take 2 four times a day, and 6 spoonfuls of the following apozem:
Guaiacum 3 oz; Sarsaparilla bark 1 oz; Sandalwood bark ½ oz; Crushed currants 3 oz; Elecampane root 1 oz; Wormwood. Boil in spring water to make up 2 pts. Take as directed.

March. As a result of taking the medicines I have prescribed for 6 weeks continuously, nearly all his symptoms had improved. I then prescribed a bitter infusion with root of

[60] Mr. Fausett was master of a ship which crossed the Irish Sea regularly, carrying coals from the Whitehaven pits to Dublin.

elecampane with other remedies for the chest. Although he denied keeping to my advice, he must have kept close to it, for his more severe symptoms cleared up and, except for a slight cough and weakness, no trace of his illness now remains.

January 7th, 1738

55 Mrs. Hale, suffering from puerperal fever, aged 30. Nine days ago she successfully gave birth. The lochia have flowed satisfactorily and are now drying up. Before delivery she suffered from an erysipeloid swelling of the face, spotted profusely by the ichorous humour. The day after delivery she had some shivering attacks, followed by a rise in temperature and very severe pain around her chest.

Signs of illness: I was called during the morning. Hard, strong, full pulse, high fever, rapid laboured breathing, severe pain throughout her chest with no sputum or cough; dry, very coated and whitish tongue, unquenchable thirst, wind in stomach, unable to sleep at all. For two days her breast milk had dried up. All other evacuating functions proceeding normally. Skin dry. Her blood was very viscous and inflamed with a large amount of serum. Her chest pain improved and her pulse slowed a little.

Diet light with copious drinks. Made a venesection in the arm and drew 10 oz of blood.
Crabs eyes 6 gr; Salt of wormwood 1 gr; Salt 1 scruple; Sugar 6 gr; Make into a powder and take 6 spoonfuls every 3 hours with this apozem:
Pectoral decoction 2 pts; Milky water 4 oz; Honey 6 scruples.

In the evening her pain became worse again and her fever returned. I prescribed an emulsion which she was unable to swallow. Her alae nasi were working.

Emulsion. Her breasts were warmed with watery milk and soap.

January 8th. A very disturbed night because of pain, and again she brought back everything she swallowed. Restless and throwing herself about. Pulse rapid, hard and of greater than normal volume. Very severe pain in all parts of her chest. 5 loose stools passed.

Blister applied to back of neck.

January 9th. Sleepless night, very restless, pulse decreased in volume but quite fast, fever and thirst less. Pain in the throat slightly less, but so far breathing has been rapid and difficult. Tongue not so dirty as before.

Hyssop water 2 oz; Mint water 2 oz; Rob. of elderflower 1 oz; Tamarind syrup 1 oz. Make a mixture. Take 1 spoonful every hour.

January 10th. Pulse harder. Other signs as before, but some troublesome vomiting.

January 11th. Slight cough.

January 12th. Fever reduced.

January 13th. Severe cough with pale copious mucoid sputum. Pulse hard and rapid. Deep respirations often achieved with great effort, producing large amounts of phlegm with a whistling sound. Severe chest pain on coughing. Bowels normal. Frequent vomiting after trying to swallow food.

January 14th. Great weakness and prostration, very rapid, weak pulse, deep respirations always with a whistling sound, increased fever with erythema of the face. Sputum less in amount. Restless.

Apply blisters to the arms.
Ammon gum ½ scruple; Pennyroyal water 6 oz; Hyssop water 6 oz; Tincture of castor 1 ½ scruples; Oxymel of squills 1 ½ oz. Take 1 spoonful every hour.

She remained in this condition until 16th January when she died about 11 o'clock in the evening.

January 5th, 1738

56 Robert Sunton, suffering from pleurisy, a sailor in his fifties and of strong fibre. On January 2nd, after he had wakened in the morning, he was first assailed by gooseflesh and a chill. This was followed by an overwhelming feeling of heat and very severe pain in his side. He had been bled on the second day of the illness and various remedies for the chest given. Two more venesections were carried out next day and on the fourth day of his illness he was bled again, but since his condition had in no way improved I was called in that day, before noon.

January 5th (4th day of illness). Signs of illness: Pulse rapid and full but not particularly hard. Very severe pain in his right side, much worse on taking a breath. Shallow, rapid, laboured breathing, slight cough which he suppressed because of the pain, with copious sputum. I prescribed an apozem and linctus.

Drink copiously of barley water flavoured with honey. Continue to use it, mixing with oxymel of squills. Take 1 spoonful every 3 hours. At midday take the apozem and linctus. Drop upon this decoction spirit of sweet salt in single doses and take barley water in a single draught. Sweet olive oil 3 oz; Syrup of marshmallow 1 ½ oz; Spirit of sulphur 20 drops; Conserve of rose hip ½ oz. Take 1 spoonful every 3 hours. Take 6 spoonfuls of this apozem: Apozem described in the *Edinburgh Pharmacopoeia* 2 pts; Nitre 3 scruples; Honey 6 scruples.
The affected parts were warmed with milky, soapy water.

In the evening the pulse was less, pain still very intense; whistling respirations because he did not want to cough or bring up material from his lungs. He was bled again from the arm and the blood was now exactly like it had been previously, with liquid serum but less inflamed. Since his bowel movements were infrequent I prescribed an emollient enema and with this, and following the venesection, his pain cleared up, his breathing became easier, and his cough looser with plentiful sputum. Tongue coated and whitish.

Drew blood in the evening. Inject an enema.

5th day of illness. Sleepless night because of coughing. He brought up large quantities of thick, dark sputum streaked with blood. Pulse fuller, pain almost completely gone, tongue moist and dusky. At night he drank ½ oz of spirit of sweet oil which I had forbidden him to take.

Pectoral decoction from the *Edinburgh Pharmacopoeia* 2 pts; Sal ammoniac 2 scruples; Oxymel of squills 1½ oz. Take 3 spoonfuls every hour, lukewarm. Shaved the hair.

6th day of illness. Weak, rapid pulse, copious, tenacious sputum, tenderness in the chest but no pain, tongue more dusky. He ate some smoked beef.

7th day of illness. Restless night because of coughing. At times his pulse was 30 per minute, at other times at the normal rate. Pustules around his mouth,[61] tongue moist but rather black, breathing less rapid and easier.

8th day of illness. Very weak pulse, great bodily weakness, breathing slower, pain still absent, very troublesome cough.

Pectoral decoction from the *Edinburgh Pharmacopoeia* 2 pts; Milky water 4 oz; Nitre ½ oz; Oxymel of squills 2 oz. Take 6 spoonfuls every 3 hours. Apply a vesicatory to the head.

For several days his cough was so bad that he was forced to sit up in a chair all night. He was coughing up a large quantity of thick phlegm. I prescribed powdered Saponac gum and other medicines for the chest. Then his feet and legs became very swollen. His chest improved and eventually in March he recovered.

January, 1738

57 Mr. Carlisle Spedding[62] a man of about 40, robust and of keen wit and sanguine temperament who from his youth had been working in the coalmining industry and is now in charge of the operations.

As a result of the suffocating vapours, he had suffered serious and lengthy spells of illness, to wit; once he was felled by the deadly vapours, and was subsequently at death's door as a result of tabes; besides this he went into the mine at the end of last summer when it was full of asphyxiating gases. His strength was hardly enough to bring him back into the daylight. Since that occasion he complained of headache and throbbing in the arteries on his head and when he thinks seriously, of a weakness in his inner sense. His breathing becomes more active, and then difficult and laboured, with a sort of constriction of his thoracic cavity. His breathing is also affected in the same way when he takes even the smallest sip of vinous spirits; if he lifts his head and face upwards, or leans backwards, he always feels dizzy. In treating these complaints I have prescribed, with no small success, these pills.

Pills formerly prescribed:
Gum ammoniac 1½ scruples; Gum galban 1½ scruples; Gum sapagen 1½ scruples; Gum myrrh 1½ scruples; Gum of aloes 1½ scruples; Venetian soap 2½ scruples; Oil of nutmeg 12 drops; Juniper oil 12 drops; Peruvian bark enough to make up pills of 5 gr. Take 3 twice a day.

January 2nd. On January 2nd, while he was walking about the tunnels of mine workings, he came to a place where water had been dammed up by a heap of earth. He

[61] Probably herpes simplex, complicating virus pneumonia with right-sided pleurisy.

[62] The brilliant mine manager in charge of all the collieries in Whitehaven. He became Brownrigg's uncle-by-marriage when the doctor married his brother's daughter. They later collaborated in experiments into the fire damp in the pits. His medical case may have arisen due to his inspection of the workings after the dreadful

crossed this place by pushing himself forward, hot and bathed in perspiration, up to his chest in the water, nor could he, in the freezing weather, change his dripping wet clothes for an hour. For two weeks afterwards he was troubled by generalized aches and pains, catarrh and other symptoms of having caught a chill.

January 15th. In the evening he had gooseflesh, a feeling of cold followed by a sensation of heat.

January 16th. Next morning I found the following signs of illness: pulse faster than normal, slight febrile heat, no difficulty in breathing, a cough which produced sharp pains in the head, persistent headache and throbbing in the head arteries, some difficulty in swallowing, whitish tongue, generalized severe pains worst in the legs, shoulders and back near the spine, a feeling of malaise and depression. The first sample of blood taken was rather inflamed.

> Diet to be light. Drew 10 oz of blood from the arm.
> Root of parsley 2 oz; Sea holly 2 scruples; Liquorice 1 oz; Tamarind ½ oz; Nitre 3 scruples; Honey ½ oz. Make a decoction in spring water up to 2 pts. Take the apozem, 6 spoonfuls warm, every 3 hours.

January 17th. Slept peacefully during the night. Increased difficulty in swallowing. Other symptoms are the same as yesterday. In the evening the headache was much worse, so I left 2 leeches applied to his temples. Then, while he was swallowing some warm whey his cough started up again and this caused the greatest difficulty in taking a breath, with a loud noise (a crowing). He attempted to clear his lungs with a tremendous effort, but for two minutes he could scarcely get any air into his chest. As a result his face turned almost black from congestion and his eyes remained fixed in a wild gaze. At last his lungs relaxed and his paroxysms of coughing ceased. For the whole of the rest of the evening he was quite lively and all his symptoms settled down fairly well.

> Decoction of barley ½ pt; Spirit of sulphur 20 drops; Rosewater 1 oz; Rose honey 2 oz. Make a gargle. Apply leeches to the temples; apply an ample blister to the shaved head.[63]

January 18th. His fever, generalized pains and headache are rather less, but his difficulty in swallowing has increased. When his throat is dry, localized pain occurs both around his larynx and the uvula which are rather inflamed. However, his appetite remains good, he is taking sugared honey drinks and milk in large amounts. At night he sweated profusely.

> Pectoral decoction from the *Edinburgh Pharmacopoeia* 2 pts. To this add between boilings: Tamarind 2 oz; Strain and add: Nitre 3 scruples; Honey 1½ oz. Make the apozem. Take 4 spoonfuls every 2 hours.

---

explosion in Corporal Pit in 1737. It was the custom for the mine overseer to inspect such dangerous works before the colliers would agree to venture down again. Later, he also suffered a broken leg, further chest trouble and severe eye damage in the course of his work. He was finally killed by an explosion in the pits in 1755. (See J. V. Beckett, 'An eighteenth-century case history: Carlisle Spedding 1738', in *Med. Hist.*, 1982, **26**: 303–6.)

[63] The remainder of this case comes after that of Mr. Rhead, but has been continued here.

January 19th. Slept deeply at intervals until his throat became dry. At one particular moment he had difficulty in inhaling. Morning: the throat infection is worse so his jugular vein had been opened and 10 oz of blood taken. The first specimen was rather inflamed.

Open the jugular vein and allow 10 oz to flow.

Evening: the inflamed areas have become very dry and he cannot swallow, so a further venesection of the arm was carried out, producing 12 oz of blood. No sign of inflammation. After being bled he did swallow. I looked at his throat and the uvula and pharynx are quite red and look inflamed.

Open the arm vein and draw 12 oz of blood.

January 20th. Slept deeply at night. No fever in the morning, but the throat is still inflamed. He has taken a draught which made him sick and he has passed five stools. While he was lying down in bed the sore throat improved, and so he lay all day on top of his bed. In the evening the sore throat was a little worse, but he can swallow without much trouble.

Leaves of senna 2 scruples; Best rhubarb 2 scruples; Tamarind 1 oz; Nitre 1½ scruples; Manna 10 scruples; Syrup of buckthorn ½ oz. Boil in spring water. Make a drink.

January 21st. Symptoms same as yesterday, except for a slight cough.

Repeat the draught. Divide with cream of tartar 6 scruples.

January 22nd. Same symptoms. He took half the prescribed medicine without vomiting, but as he could not swallow the rest without feeling sick, I prescribed cream of tartar to be taken on 3 occasions, resulting in seven stools. Sore throat slightly better.

Mucilage made from quince seed 8 oz; Rose water 1 oz; Sal Prunella 1½ scruples; Honey 1 oz. Make a gargle.

January 24th. As his bowels have not moved for 2 days, and he was unwilling to take the laxative draught again, I ordered an enema which produced 2 stools. He is swallowing more easily and is sitting up nearly all day, without much effort. Profuse sweating at night.

Rhubarb 1 scruple; Salt of wormwood 6 gr; Boil in spring water and make up 3 oz. Strain and add: Root of Mexican bindweed 1 scruple; Rose syrup 3 scruples; Spirit of lavender ½ scruple.

January 25th. I prescribed a laxative medicine—result 5 stools. Tongue looks rather dirty and almost black. Rather painful cough and a sort of catarrh in the chest with head pains which are particularly sharp in the left temple.

January 26th. On examining the throat, the uvula appeared normal, but on the posterior part of the pharynx and upper part of the larynx can be seen diffuse white spots looking like bacon or rather a crust of aphthae, yet the pain and difficulty in swallowing have decreased. These ulcers on his throat gradually cleared up but his wrists, knees and ankles remained affected by rheumatic pains until almost the end of April. These joints were also rather weak and his wrists and ankles often swelled up, but all the other symptoms of his illness completely disappeared, nor did he have any more trouble with headaches or chest symptoms. Indeed he enjoyed better health than before he was taken ill.

January, 1738

58 Mr. Rhead,[64] the famous artist. A man of about 70, thin and of a melancholy temperament, living a very temperate lifestyle, of a keen wit and utterly wrapped up in his work. For most of his life he had had no illnesses with the exception of gout, but his attacks of this disease had been only slight, and rarely invasive. However, being intolerant of pain, five years ago he wanted to avoid this problem by taking cold baths. As a result his pain promptly came back and the skin on his legs was raised into vesicles full of fluid. The vesicles shed the fluid and healed up in a short time. The gout hardly troubled him until the end of last summer when he avoided the pain by the same method, but a little while later—within a few days in fact—he was tormented by the most dreadful colicky abdominal pain, accompanied by vomiting. The pains extended all over the right side, from the pubis up to the lower ribs. By using opiates, oily and diuretic draughts, and turpentine enemas and venesection, the pains were relieved on these occasions, or perhaps more often.

N.B.: The first time he used cold baths following the attack his legs were swollen, but the second time he did this as the attack began.

January 13th. Now, because of a chill he had caught, the pains returned afresh with increased violence, for on 13th of this month in the afternoon they assailed the wretched man in the same part of his body. At the beginning of the attack he vomited a great deal and his pain returned frequently.

January 15th. During the night following 15th the pain was extremely severe, and next morning I was sent for. The remedies he had been taking were tried out with no effect.

January 16th. Signs of illness: Strong, slow, regular, hard pulse, abdomen swollen and tense. At every moment the most cruel pains were extending throughout the whole length of the colon on the right side as if his bowels were being pierced by a gimlet. He was moaning and groaning continually. No signs of stones or gravel. A small stool was produced after a clyster. In the evening his pain settled fairly well.

> Common decoction 14 oz; Olive oil 2 oz. Make a clyster. Mallow leaves 2 oz; Marshmallow leaves 2 oz; Root of sea holly 2 scruples; Root of liquorice 1 oz; Manna 1 oz; Honey ½ oz. Make an apozem. 4 spoonfuls to be swallowed warm every hour.

January 17th. At 11 p.m. the pains returned and lasted all night, but not so severely as on the previous night. The pains were always relieved by a clyster, but once the clyster was returned the pains troubled him sorely again.

> Repeat the clyster.

[64] Rhead (or Read) was the most famous artist in Whitehaven. Under the patronage of Sir James Lowther and the merchants of the town he executed portraits, several "bird's eye" views of Whitehaven, and painted panels in houses and churches. In leaner periods he also decorated rooms at the Flatt, and painted the Newcomen engine at Saltom Pit. He died on 8th November 1747, aged 78, and was buried in Holy Trinity church.

Sometimes the pains extended to the whole length of his back, up to the back of his neck; at others they were felt between the innominate bones. No abdominal swelling.

11 in the morning. Gave a clyster and repeated at 3 p.m. Warm the feet with warm water and apply a blistering plaster of equal parts and an epispastic for the head.

January 18th to 22nd. During the whole of this period the pains were rather less and often completely absent. However, they did trouble him fairly severely twice. Once during the night following 18th, the pain started about 2 a.m. and lasted for eight hours when a paroxysm remitted and he felt arthritic pain in his knees. He removed the poultice from his feet. On the 20th, after a meal of sweet oranges, the pain once again assailed him most cruelly with spasms of the abdominal muscles. After four or five hours I prescribed a clyster. Immediately after this was administered the pain remitted. He returned a large quantity of faeces and flatus with the enema fluid and the pain was much improved, but as was his habit, he remained in very low spirits throughout the attack and then again burst out suddenly with a groan.

On the 18th I prescribed a draught with a Matthew's pill of 15 gr.
On the 19th I prescribed another drink of a soothing draught. Warmed the affected parts with an apozem of herbs and seeds warmed, with which the wind was removed and the pain remitted.
Emollient decoction 10 oz; Venetian turpentine ½ oz; Sweet olive oil 1½ oz. Use footbaths repeatedly every day and rub his feet. Diet should be of easily digestible foods with white wine and beer.

On the 21st in the evening, his stomach was distended; he was very depressed and the arthritic pains in his knees and ankles came back. Abdominal colic affected the poor man all night, but rather less severely than previously. In the morning he was again free from abdominal colic and the arthritic pain had once more localized in his ankle. This morning, that is January 22nd, I have prescribed some pills. Bowels moving once a day. Belching up a lot of wind.

Gum of sagapenum 2 scruples; Gum opopanax 2 scruples; Gum of myrrh 2 scruples; Extract of liquorice 2 scruples; Castor 2 scruples; Saffron 2 scruples; Oil of aniseed 12 drops; Juniper 12 drops; Balsam of copaiba, enough to make pills of 6 gr. Take 2 four times every day with 3 spoonfuls of white wine.

March 28th. For three or four hours he was again racked by very severe pain in the right iliac area. Next day he passed two stones the size of large peas per urethram.[65]

January 26th, 1738

59 Master Jonathan Kelsick, a boy of 11, of poor constitution. On January 26th, in the afternoon, he was suddenly taken ill with a fever, accompanied by a severe headache which became worse during the night, and he also developed a pain in his side.

[65] Brownrigg considered a diagnosis of right sided renal colic here, as he states "no signs of stones or gravel", but as the patient did not produce any such clinical evidence the doctor was diverted to the incorrect diagnosis of intestinal disease, possibly recurrent sub-acute obstruction, until almost three months later when Mr. Rhead passed two moderate-sized stones per urethram.

January 27th. Next morning, Mr. Smith bled him from the arm and the blood was inflammatory with much densely coagulated serum. In the evening I was sent for.

Signs of illness: Pulse fluttering hard, bounding and rapid, fast laboured breathing, slight cough suppressed because of pain, bowels open, tongue moist and whitish, black sores around mouth and teeth, not much thirst, no appetite, pain in the right side towards the back which was hurting him considerably. He lies in a coma and is delirious on waking. He turns away all medicaments by mouth. Skin dry and hot. In the evening the blood was less inflamed than in the morning.

Morning. 6 oz of blood was taken. Let diet be light and diluting.
Evening. 6 oz of blood was taken again.
11 p.m. Applied a blistering plaster the size of a nut.

January 28th. Quite a peaceful night. Fever just as high as before, but no pain in the side. Seems to be quite confused in his mind although responding at first, but he rolls his eyes. Breathing easier than yesterday, skin dry, no strangury from vesicatories, urine whitish and turbid, almost like mucus, nostrils working, tongue coated and tending somewhat to be dusky in colour, but moist. Blood is just as inflamed as on the first occasion. Towards night he is delirious at times and cannot tolerate the slightest noise.

Use common linctus when wanted. Drink copiously from a cold emulsion. At 4 p.m. take 6 oz of blood again.

January 29th. Night time extremely restless, hardly any sleep. In the morning, pulse strong and hard, but less so than yesterday, skin not so hot as yesterday but still dry, nostrils working. Slept for 2 hours. About midday, when he awoke, I found his pulse to be rapid and feeble, yet hard, so I ordered a plaster to be applied to his feet. After this was done he was very anxious and miserable during the whole afternoon and was really worried lest vesicatories should be applied to his feet. On examining the patient at 5 p.m. I found pulse rapid, weak, and a little harder than at midday, skin slightly moist, breathing quite rapid and shallow, cough considerably checked but no complaint of pain. After I had assured him that the plaster would produce only slight blisters, practically all his symptoms settled down. Bowels moved twice today.

Blister the head with an epispastic in equal parts. Apply a plaster to the feet.

January 30th. Night: restless; sleep quite disturbed.

Morning: Bled 2 oz. Pulse almost normal but a little hard, laboured breathing, nostrils working, suppressing the cough less than yesterday. Dirty tongue. For the whole of today he has slept peacefully, breathing much easier. In the evening he coughs with some effort a clear mucoid sputum. Urine straw-coloured without sediment. Has passed hard faeces like a wide worm.

Morning. Take 2 oz of blood.

January 31st. Night—slept at intervals. Pulse slow, regular, of normal volume, slightly hard, no fever, cough and mucoid sputum, breathing easier and slower, but shallow, appetite returning, often bathed in profuse perspiration.

Sweet almond oil; Syrup; Balsam; Violet; Peruvian bark ½ scruple; Yolk of egg 3 scruples. Make a linctus. Take a level spoonful every 2 hours.

February 1st. Pulse quite slow, regular and strong, no fever, breathing regular and easy with no cough, appetite improving. The illness has quite cleared up and only a feeling of weakness remains.

February 19th, 1738

60 Mr. Jonathan Carlyle, a merchant, a young man aged 19, obese and of good bodily constitution. For one week he had been suffering from diarrhoea and catarrh with a slight cough, and during this time, for three consecutive days, he had been indulging in strenuous dancing until 3 o'clock in the morning. Then, hot and sweating he had ventured into the keen cold of an icy night. Next day the frost had gone. Yesterday evening he suddenly became dizzy, a book fell from his hands and he could hardly hold himself up in his chair. He felt very hot all through the night, he was parched, throwing his arms and legs about from one place to another in bed. During his sleep he was talking a great deal of nonsense and was sweating copiously. This morning, signs of illness: weak, rapid, regular pulse, very high fever, dry skin, rapid laboured breathing, slight cough with thin sputum often mixed with streaks of blood, tongue whitish and moist, tremendous thirst, a feeling of malaise, utter prostration, dizziness and generalised head and chest pains, somewhat aggravated by coughing, with lancinating pain in the head and the right side. Body heat becomes intense at times. Nature of the illness: a fever epidemic in this type of constitution. In order to alleviate it I started off the following regime. Blood looks perfectly healthy. 3 stools today.

February 19th. Morning. Take 10 oz of blood from the arm.
Elderflower water 3 oz; Weak cinnamon water 3 oz; Vitriolated tartar 1½ scruples; Nitre 1½ scruples; Rob. of elderflower 2 oz. Take 1 spoonful every 2 hours.
Evening. Apply a blistering plaster to the back of the neck. Cucumber seed 1 oz; White poppy seed ½ oz; Sweet almond oil No. 15; 2 pts spring water; Rose water 1 oz; Hollyhock syrup 1½ oz. Make an emulsion.

February 20th. Morning—pulse so weak that my finger could scarcely feel it. Showing huge blisters as a result of the epispastics, no strangury, remaining symptoms as before. Turbid urine. Evening—bowels moved 7 times, pulse stronger, headache and vertigo almost gone. He appears more lively.

Senna 2 scruples; Tamarind 1 oz; Rhubarb 2 scruples; Nitre 1½ scruples; Manna 1 oz. Boil in spring water to make up 4 oz. Take in the morning.

February 21st. Night—restless, disturbed sleep without relief. Pulse fairly strong, but fast. More pain in the side.

Take this anodyne draught with 6 scruples of diacod, nitre and spermaceti.

February 22nd. Pulse very fast and weak, unproductive cough without sputum, pain much less but no diarrhoea. The anodyne was repeated. Thereafter by means of a few other remedies, he recovered from his attack over the space of 3 or 4 days.

Take 10 oz of blood.
Fennel root 2 oz; Parsley 2 oz; Liquiorice 1 oz; Coltsfoot 1 oz; Hollyhock 1 oz; Nitre 3 scruples; Rob. of elderflower 1 ½ oz. Make the apozem. Take 4 spoonfuls every hour.

May 3rd, 1738

61 The Reverend Mr. Sewel,[66] aged 28 years, a man of keen wit, wrapped up in his literary studies and nocturnal readings. Perhaps he indulges too much in alcoholic liquors, as they say, to keep up his spirits when depressed. In other respects he is a temperate, sober man. He has suffered for many years from an intermittent fever which he had suppressed too often and unreasonably with Peruvian bark and has had recourse to it so often that he used to eat it greedily when at his books. The fever has ceased for two years, yet there remains cachexia, skinniness and bodily prostration. This spring after he had been studying too much during the night, and serious mental affections, the following symptoms were seen: pulse quite irregular, which is diagnostic of great weakness of vital forces, no appetite, after meals he develops heat and redness of the face. After deep thought he often becomes dizzy and there arises some anaesthesia. His bowels remain constipated for 7 days. Hoarseness of voice often attacks him suddenly, yet it always clears up again quickly. A scirrhous swelling has appeared between the lower jaw and the ear on the right side.

See the consultation with Boerhaave on page . . .[67]
Root of hyssop 1 ½ oz; Root of American mulberry 2 oz; Virginian snake root 2 oz; Wormwood 3 scruples. Pour into 2 pts of old Rhenish wine, strain and take 3 spoonfuls an hour before breakfast, lunch and dinner every day. A draught of whey or milk stout.
Pill Ruffus 2 scruples; Castor 2 scruples; Borax 15 gr; Peruvian bark, enough to make up 30 pills, 2 of which should be swallowed at one dose at night at bedtime, so that the bowels respond once in the day.

February 17th, 1741[68]

Still cachectic and thin with great bodily prostration. His digestion and strength truly broken down by weakness. He has a dropsical swelling of the legs which occurs nearly every year and is especially troublesome in the spring, but there is no fever or thirst or urinary problem.

Root of zedoary 2 scruples; Myrrh extract 6 scruples; Crocus of iron 1 ½ scruples; Type of Diamber 1 ½ oz; Yellow saffron 1 ½ oz; Syrup of clove pink. Take the amount of a nutmeg at 10 a.m. and 5 p.m. every day. In addition take 4 spoonfuls of: Shaved sassafras wood 1 ½ oz; Red sandalwood shavings 3 scruples; Root of angelica 3 scruples; Hyssop 3 scruples; Elecampane 3 scruples; Gentian 2 scruples; Juniper berry 2 oz; Cream of tartar 1 scruple. Boil in a closed container for 1 ½ hrs in spring water to make up 2 pts. Add to the boiling liquid: Leaves of horseradish 2 oz. Leave to settle for 4 hrs; strain and add: Strong cinnamon water 2 oz.

[66] Minister of Holy Trinity church. After this illness he kept his church death record complete with causes of death from 1751 until his death in 1780. As this is an unusual occurrence, perhaps he was influenced by Brownrigg.

[67] This has not been included in the Casebook.

[68] A later insert.

May 10th, 1738

62 Mrs. Holmes, a widow in the clothing trade, much given to hysterical affections, 45 years old with a spotty complexion, slow, and always suffering from some complaint or other. On May 5th she took a purgative draught, as is her custom almost every spring. On May 6th blood was taken from her arm. On the 8th she took another stronger laxative draught, with the result that she moved her bowels 12 times. Next night she had a lot of vomiting and diarrhoea. She became quite ill and feverish. Towards evening she vomited again and her bowels moved 5 or 6 times. She fell ill and was sick all night, and so next morning I was called in.

The last draught was made up of: Senna ½ oz; boiled in water with cream of tartar and cardamom seed. Rose syrup was then added to the solution.

May 10th. Signs of illness: Pulse rapid and rather hard, feverish, whitish coated moist tongue. A wakeful coma, for she has a tendency to sleep most of the time, but when she first went to sleep she was often aroused by huge stomach pains, anxiety and feeling ill, which settled again after she had been sick. In addition, she has had her menstrual period for 2 days.

Tamarind 1 oz; Cream of tartar ½ oz; Iris root 1 scruple; Cardamom seed 1 scruple. Boil and add cream of tartar in solution to make up 1 pt. Add this to the decoction while boiling and also dissolve 10 scruples of manna. Strain and add strong cinnamon water 2 oz. Take 6 spoonfuls every hour.

May 13th. After taking the decoction she has improved markedly, however there remains slight fever which becomes worse now and again and which last night occurred with greater force. The fever is accompanied by very severe pain in her side, and stomach pain, thirst, nausea and anxiety with palpitations. Today, all these symptoms have settled down. Pulse weak and regular but a little faster. Her menstrual period has now completely finished.

Take blood from arm 6 oz.
Black barley water 2 oz; Pennyroyal water 2 oz; Bryony water 1 oz; Treacle water 1 oz; Spirit of lavender 2 scruples; Tincture of castor 2 scruples; Tincture of saffron 2 scruples; Tartar of vitriol 1 scruple; Sugar 3 scruples. Make a julep and take 2 spoonfuls every hour.

May 14th. Slept well at night, nor have her symptoms returned except that she has slight abdominal pain from time to time. She is depressed and has other hysterical symptoms.

About April, 1738

63 Mrs. Pool, a woman of 46 with a tendency to mental affections and poor digestion, also suffering from oedematous swellings of the knees. After many episodes of weeping she eventually developed excessive menstrual bleeding, a complaint from which she had quite often suffered before and which caused bad digestion and swellings. When I was called in she had already had vaginal bleeding for a whole month, although meanwhile Dr. H. had treated her with large quantities of binding medicine in a powder, which made her constipated. She was quite prostrate with weakness due to the excessive loss, so that she was unable to leave her bed.

Some observations drawn from this case.
Powdered restringents made from coral. A bolus and similar remedies.

Her pulse was very weak. She was feeling low and very much depressed by fear and anxiety. From time to time she felt a kind of crawling of the flesh or a pressure of all the humours of the body upwards and downwards upon her womb. After a short time a large flow of florid blood poured vigorously from her vagina. At first I treated her with a 50 gr bolus of rhubarb and one drop of oil of cinnamon. This produced 2 bowel motions. At bedtime I prescribed opiates to diminish the blood loss, but although she had not slept previously and the loss was made worse by throwing herself about, yet she was hardly any better while asleep because of the fever and increased blood flow caused by the opium. Every now and then, both while asleep and as soon as she awoke, the blood poured forth in greater amounts than ever. I then prescribed the decanted remedy of Septalius[69] so much praised by Dr. Woodhouse, senior: to wit: Peel of orange, to which I added pomegranate bark, red roses, spirits of vitriol and other substances to stem the flow of blood, yet for 2 days the illness did not yield to treatment with these preparations. On applying linen cloths soaked in vinegar to the hypogastrium and the vagina, the bleeding was always decreased to some extent, and this regime was continued during the whole course of the treatment. Then I ordered nettle juice, ½ oz to be taken hourly, and I applied large cupping glasses to her breasts two or three times daily and ligatures to her arms and thighs. She continued to take the nettle juice for 3 days and the bleeding diminished a little with this and with the application of the other remedies. She then took 15 drops of spirit of vitriol every 2 hours for four or five days, and afterwards. Tincture Antiphthisica, and so at last, within twelve days from the time I had first been called in, the bleeding completely stopped.

1738

64 Mr. Lamplugh Simpson, dry gangrene of the stomach. A lawyer, an inhabitant of Cockermouth, aged 26. He is much given to drinking beer and ale, and because of this, and his sedentary lifestyle, he is of an obese and leucophlegmatic disposition. For eighteen months he has had upper abdominal swelling and stomach pains, and after drinking he suffers from very violent copious vomiting of blood and purulent material. As a result he has often been at death's door, afterwards often experiencing slight rigors from the same cause.

June 4th. On 4th June, 1738, as he was intending to marry on 6th, he set off for Whitehaven to obtain the ecclesiastical licence. Before he had left home he was seized by very severe stomach pains and to relieve these he took 1½ oz of rhubarb medicine. During the journey he could not bear the discomfort of being shaken by the motion of his horse, and so travelled the greater part of the way slowly on foot, and in order to relieve his insatiable thirst and his pain, he swallowed strong ales, gin and white wine in large amounts. After spending 6 whole hours on the journey, he at last reached Whitehaven weary and exhausted by illness. About 4 o'clock in the afternoon I was called to see him and observe the following signs:

[69] Obviously a well-tried remedy of Septalius.

Rapid, hard pulse, very high fever, severe thirst, tongue whitish and dry, acute pain in the region of the stomach, abdominal swelling enormous. He felt extremely ill. I prescribed a draught of Riverius[70] with 10 drops of liquid laudanum in the evening, which he vomited back. After this he concluded his business, and about 9 p.m. he was bled, 10 oz from his arm. The blood appeared slightly inflamed. He then vomited again, so in order to relieve his stomach I tried gruels, milk stout, green tea and similar bland fluids, and later I repeated the draught with 20 drops of liquid laudanum, but he vomited this back too. Indeed he never stopped vomiting all night.

June 5th. Early morning, about 4 a.m., I was sent for and found a full, strong, rapid pulse, hot prickly skin, great anxiety and prostration, dusky tongue and unquenchable thirst. The vomit now appeared black in colour, like coffee grounds; his stomach was grossly distended. He had difficulty in swallowing, and most of what he swallowed was sticking to the upper entrance to the stomach. His breath seemed to catch in his throat and he had frequent fears of suffocation, so that he was often obliged to try and make himself sick by putting his fingers down his throat. I bled him again, 10 oz, and the blood looked more inflamed than what I had taken previously. I then gave him a cathartic and his bowels moved once. I again tried a thin soup of chicken and oats, and this he returned mixed with dark bile-coloured material. I gave him 30 or 40 drops of liquid laudanum from a spoon and some of Riverius' julep. He vomited back one dose of the first and I tried the other, but the sickness did not stop with this method, although in the course of 5 hours I had tried him with 2 oz of liquid laudanum. In addition the enema was repeated 4 or 5 times. Meanwhile the pain was still severe and he still had the thirst, the anxiety and the other symptoms. With every hour his pulse became weaker, more rapid and more irregular. At about the first hour of the afternoon the venesection was repeated and the blood was very inflamed. I also applied a poultice of treacle mixed with turpentine to his abdomen. About 3 p.m. he vomited material which appeared to be what he had swallowed. About 5 p.m. the vomiting and pain stopped, so that I began to have great hopes that he would recover. But his pulse was extremely irregular, small and very weak, his extremities were very cold, and he remained quiet but could not sleep till 1 a.m.

June 6th. Very weak. His fiancée then arrived. He was delighted to see her and had a short talk with her. He told her he was much better, however his conversation showed some slight mental confusion. His fiancée had hardly left his bedside when after tossing and turning, he died within two minutes.

No opportunity was given to perform an autopsy.[71]

June 4th, 1738

65 Joyce Peel, Mr. Clementson's niece, a single girl aged 18. She was seized by fever and vomiting, severe pains in the stomach and bowels and on passing her motions. Mr. Clementson bled her, and on June 5th he treated her with a purgative medicine. On the seventh day I was called in and found: rapid, weak, irregular pulse, vomiting and pains settled. I bled her and treated her with an opening apozem. Her blood was slightly inflamed.

[70] A remedy prescribed by Lazare Rivière (1589–1655).

[71] This 26-year-old man was an alcoholic. The chronic gastric inflammation which often accompanied this condition no doubt caused the repeated vomiting of dark coffee ground material. The patient's own

9th day shivering attacks with very weak pulse. I applied a cupping glass to the back of her neck and prescribed Riverius' julep and emulsions with clysters as required.

10th day more shivering attacks with jerking of the tendons.

11th day. Her symptoms were much improved, but I applied two vesicatories to her legs first thing in the morning. A short time afterwards the fever cleared up.

66 Mrs. James Milham,[72] inflammation of the intestines. A pretty young woman of 18 with a beautiful complexion and dainty figure, who was in the eighth month of her first pregnancy. About her fifth month, after a spell of frosty weather, she suffered from a purplish erysipeloid fever (a rash fever) which disappeared leaving no trace despite no evacuative means being applied. However, she was left with a very troublesome cough which affected her particularly at night time, and she often suffered excruciating pain in her lower back.

On 1st June she had sat all afternoon in a damp, cold place. On 5th June, about 4 a.m., she was seized with severe pains in the stomach, vomited several times and moved her bowels four or five times. At 9 a.m. I found full, rapid pulse, distended veins. Her pains were very severe and her cries could be heard a long way away. I treated her with large doses of liquid laudanum, giving it 4 or 5 times after each episode of vomiting, but the pain was only a little relieved by this regime. About 11 a.m. I bled her of 17 oz of blood which looked inflamed. I then gave her further doses of laudanum and applied a poultice of Andromachus treacle, breadcrumbs and red wine to her abdomen. With this treatment the pain settled, but her backache and fever remained. On June 7th she was bled again. After this she gradually recovered and gave birth to a healthy infant.[73]

SKIN DISEASES

On skin rashes.

Definition of a rash. The tumours of a rash are scanty and hard, especially when occurring on the face. After they have suppurated they disappear (a). The Greeks call them 'ἴονθοι.

Nature of rashes. Therefore these spots are small areas of phlegmonous humour which go on to laudable pus, and are situated in the papillary vessels of the skin and in the exhaling cutaneous arteries, whence they leave no scar.

First type. This condition is hereditary in many people, mostly in the fleshy parts, to wit, the face; it then spreads to the arms, buttocks and chest. It comes to a climax at the beginning of the third week and disappears spontaneously at the end of the fifth week. It is aggravated by catching cold or by any other abnormality in the normal course of events, especially the excessive use of spirituous liquors or even drinking water.

---

treatment—more alcohol—and Brownrigg's administration of laudanum were both inappropriate, as Simpson might have been suffering from liver disease (cirrhosis) resulting from his drinking habits.

[72] Wife of James Milham, a merchant with ships engaged in the Virginia trade. Formerly Miss Isabella Kelsick, she had been married in St. Nicholas church on 15 February 1736. She died in August 1741.

[73] Cases 64, 65, and 66 are tightly grouped on two pages. It seems that Brownrigg was linking them in respect of the sudden onset of stomach pains.

Second type. Another type of this condition results from retention of some normal outflow of blood. For instance, from staunching a nosebleed according to Actuarius, or is common in a woman whose menstruation is in some way improper, for I have observed a rash breaking out about the time of a monthly period, and it particularly affects the arms. Yet as soon as the period is over it goes away without suppurating (b). Women at the end of the third month of pregnancy are often affected by spots which mainly occur on the face and last throughout lactation. They disappear completely as soon as the monthly periods start again (c).

(a) According to Galen, Actuarius, Aetius, Paul of Aegina, etc. See Sebizius 'Medical Mirror', Vol. I, p. 415.[74]

(b) As I have observed in Mr. Ritson's daughter, and in my own sister Nicholson.

(c) Mrs. Dean suffered from this type of skin rash.

SKIN DISEASES: THE VARIOUS TYPES OR RASHES

Proximate causes of rashes. The first type of skin rash is seen to arise from the natural fabric of the body, and especially from any fault of the over-relaxed solid tissues, whence the static humours are driven into the cutaneous arteries, their wrong place, and create inflammation there. Indeed this condition is well known to occur in young people—so perhaps plethora should be joined to the first cause. It is aggravated by any cause which induces an inflammatory diathesis in the humours.

The second type depends on the plethora.[75]

Treatment. Many consider this illness to be due to sharp and thick humours and they call it Scurvy. I know by experience moreover this condition is wrongly treated by purges, cures, and other warm refined antiscorbutics, sal volatile and such like. The first type are suited by strengthening digestive remedies which develop all the natural excretions, e.g.: a digestible diet, gum pills with soap. Fontanels and vesicatories are also helpful. The second type are suited by whatever moves blocked humours, and in pregnant women, what removes the plethora but maintains their strength. In all types, fatty and indigestible cooked foods are to be avoided, but all suffer with cold or excess heat. They are able to benefit from rubbing and exercises, particularly on horseback.

Aetius in Book No. 8, Chapter 13,[76] and other ancient writers have recommended various other types of emollient, topical remedies, dispersants and cleansers.

ON IMPETIGO OR THE GREEK LEPROSY

February 19th, 1738

67 Matthew Rotchford's son, a youth aged 17, a barber. He was of a sanguine constitution and somewhat softer fibre. After taking frequent cold baths 2 years ago he developed impetigo. Many spots appeared, first on his head, jaws and forearms, then all over the rest of his skin. There developed purplish-white desquamations. When these flakes peeled off, the skin underneath was red and later became hard with flaky crusts. Dr. Senhouse prescribed purgatives, then various other remedies, first mercurial preparations, then warm baths. After the baths, the flaky eruptions spread all over his whole body, but on treating

[74] Melchior Sebizius, *Manualis sive speculum medicinae*, Strassburg, F. Spoor, 1661.

[75] A bodily condition, or an excess of blood.

[76] Aetius Amidenus, *De cognoscendis et curandis morbis*, Basle, 1533.

him with sorrel ointment they at last disappeared. But, they troubled him again at about the same time of the spring equinox every year. This spring (1738) he used Plummer's Pills for a whole month which are described as follows in the *Medical Essays*, Vol. I:[77]

> Golden sulphur; Antimony Salts of Angelica 3 parts; Calomel 2 parts; or for a stronger mixture, grind and crush them both together in a mortar with sufficient extract of gentian and drops of clove pink oil. Then make a pill so that the patient takes 15 gr of the powder described daily, in divided doses, morning and evening.

The above powder first acts by increasing insensible perspiration. After a cold at the time of taking it, slight excessive salivation was caused. On taking 10 gr on an empty stomach in the morning he felt sick, vomited a little, and moved his bowels once. Having taken this treatment himself for a month, Plummer, its inventor, cured dandruff which was spreading in hard crusts all over his forehead and this had failed to respond to calomel, antiscorbutics, liniments and lotions. Once the excessive salivation had been stimulated, the crusts went away for four or five months, but they returned with equal severity the next spring.

A person aged 24 had considerable foulness of the face from many red spots and pimples, as this eruption happened suddenly upon taking cold; bleedings, blisterings and frequent purges were tried in the beginning, but with little advantage. Afterwards antiscorbutic juices, Gum pills with soap, medicated whey and goat whey were used for a considerable time with no better success, and at length even six weeks salivation failed of removing these obstinate Pimples. In the space of two months these were carried off by the Use of the remedy aforesaid, with the assistance only of a gently drying and detergent lotion towards the End of the Cure.[78] Plummer, ibidem.

Mr. Davidson (during my visit to Carlisle), a man of 30, of sanguine constitution, agile and robust and of a sprightly disposition, took a copious draught of an ice-cold drink while he was very much heated by the chase. Within a few days some superficial spots broke out on his face, somewhat dusky in colour, as I recall, in sparse groups which then progressed to large maculae, producing thin fluid and peeling off to form purplish flakes of skin. These same maculae appeared on his arms and all over his body. To clear these up he used mineral water from Moffat, and this having no result, expelled pus, however the spots did not respond. He went to London and there underwent a long and expensive course of drying liquors, venesection, emetics, cathartics and hot baths, which were no more successful than his previous treatment.

Practically all the Milham family of this town were affected by impetigo, such as was described in the case of the barber. Nothing availed against this illness, not purgatives, antiscorbutics, salivations as shown by repeated experiences. They found, however, that of all the ointment in Willis's *Pharmacopoeia* (Part 2, page 423)[79] the following one was outstandingly successful:

[77] Andrew Plummer, 'An alternative mercurial medicine', *Medical Essays and Observations*, issued by the Philosophical Society of Edinburgh, T. and W. Ruddimans, 1733, vol. 1, pp. 46–62.

[78] Ibid., pp. 56–7.

[79] Thomas Willis, *Pharmaceutice rationalis*, vol. 1, The Hague, A. Leers, 1677, p. 515.

> Take a portion of fatty meat from a wether and place it in a vessel. Over a period of time gradually soak it by continually adding drops of liquid tar, and the substance which collects at the bottom of the vessel can be used as an ointment. It makes the skin smooth again and washes away the flakes of skin remarkably well.

Mr. Milham and Mr. Coates, after salivations and other unsuccessful remedies, were cured by Scarborough water.[80]

Willis—On Impetigo or Greek Leprosy in his *Pharmacopoeia Rat.*, Vol. I, part 2.[81] "The preceding causes of these diseases are fatty, salty and indigestible food such as pork, fish (especially shellfish), scurvy and venereal disease. This condition is commonest among the inhabitants of coastal resorts and marshy places. Many newborn babies with quite severe impetigo have travelled to our spa waters in Bath, whence they have returned with true leprosy". These are the author's very words.

Salivation cures impetigo temporarily, but unless the disease has developed from a venereal infection, it returns afterwards with even greater disfigurement. The author states this with emphasis, giving many examples.

N.B.: The same author warns that even after confidently using salivations as a cure and at the same time completely healing the disease with mercury purgatives for a month, along with sweatings and a diet of decoctions of sarsaparilla and tea, etc. nevertheless the disease is just like the Hydra: when one head is cut off, it comes back to life sevenfold.

The measures most acclaimed for the condition are: venesection and especially purgatives with rhubarb and sorrel; whey with chalybeate waters; juice extracted from succulent herbs, especially chicory and dandelions; decoctions of bark; meat extracts with ferruginous waters are often helpful remedies. Indeed, when all other treatments have failed, with these alone I have several times cured severe and almost leprous impetigo. For violent itchings and persistent skin eruptions, Sydenham has used sudorifics. H.S. a liquid posset to be drunk each morning, and the application of Oxylap ointment to the affected parts. For dandruff he recommends an ointment containing ashes of leaves and wood. I recall Boerhaave prescribed, inter alia, for Dr. Hutton, for dandruff, tobacco leaves soaked in vinegar to be applied to the area. Horstius has written the following account of what he calls obstinate sores which went on to become Greek leprosy: Vol. 2, p. 341.[82]

"A country youth aged 15 years had suffered from early childhood from a dry, scabby skin, peeling off purplish flakes of shrivelled skin with alterating induration, being left with a truly appalling appearance. Principles of management: 1. To drive away noxious humours through the bowels. 2. To soften and remove completely the rooted, affected areas of skin. 3. To strengthen nature to prevent a return of the condition. With respect to the first principle, Hydromel laxative was used for eight days, together with rhubarb, agric, senna, sorrel, chicory, fumitory, etc. For the second, he used baths containing bryony root, sorrel, lime, active sulphur, etc., and afterwards a liniment made up of the same substances, also goats' whey as a laxative with senna and chicory, fumitory, dandelion, etc., followed by sudorifics made from elderflower, sambucus and mithridatum and yellow sulphur diaphoretics. With these few remedies continued over a period of three

[80] A later insertion.
[81] Ibid., pp. 495–518.
[82] Gregor Horst, *Opera medica*, 3 vols, Gouda, G. van der Hoeve, 1661.

weeks, the patient was fully restored to health and was still alive and well three years later. With respect to the third principle, for 3 days a week he used Hydromel laxative with a conserve of fumitory and chicory root and in the second year I advised him to take a cure at Bad Geissingen".

Platter uses the same methods. Moreover, he writes of two other similar striking successes.

Elephantiasis as described by Aretaeus differs as much from the Greek leprosy as from the leprosy of the Jews and Arabs. Often the disease is hereditary and is caught either by contagion or spontaneously by personal default. Throughout the ages it has been asserted to be incurable and so lepers have everywhere been segregated from society.[83] The disease is as frequent in hot regions like Alexandria as in colder northern areas such as France and Germany (although Lucretius denies this: the elephantine disease, which arises because of the River Nile in the middle of Egypt, never spreads any further). Forestus states that there are many elephantiasis cases in Batavia, where the atmosphere is heavy and humid (as in Alexandria) on account of using salt meat and bad pickled fish and fish which has not been well salted. By the same reasoning, Willis argues that this disease was indeed well known to the Cornish. At all events, in different areas the disease itself has different symptoms. Duretus' commentary on Hollerus [*sic*]:[84] The first stage is intractable alphos. This is followed by ringworm and eruptions which together involve roughness and itching and often prickliness. After the eruptions come the "Psora" which Hippocrates calls "bran" in his book on Diet.[85] The Psora turn into leprosy and when this is present, the fore areas are truly thickened with deep, bleeding ulcers. From leprous areas the condition goes on to elephantiasis itself, or generalised cancer. Riverius tells of the following cases:[86]

"A certain woman, a fisherwoman whose husband had died of Leprosy, was suffering from impetigo all over her body with so much itching that she constantly scratched herself. In the mornings, because of her ceaseless scratching, three or four pecks of skin flakes collected in her bed, like so many fishscales. Having been ordered a bland diet, laxatives with cassia and venesection, then a magistral syrup with rhubarb, millipede, senna, etc., and keeping her bowels open for 30 days, at the same time taking whey and then the waters of *Meiningen*,[87] the patient was restored to perfect health, nor did she require my services for 15 years afterwards. The waters of *Meiningen* are vitriolated waters" (ibid., p. 318). "A boy of ten suffering from impetigo was sweating a watery discharge. This foul material was suppressed by successive west winds and turned to his lungs, which brought about an appalling attack of asthma. This stopped immediately by a disposition of warm winds."

Rondelet, in Scholz *Consilia et Epistolae* p. 842:[88] "Women, boys and eunuchs rarely suffer from elephantiasis. These people are of a more moist humour and the moisture itself resists drying out. Aetius says that many men have protected themselves from this disease by castration. By this means I freed a youth this year who had started with the disease and moreover had progressed beyond the early stages."

[83] *Idem*, 'Examination of lepers', ibid., p. 345.
[84] Jacobus Hollerius, *Opera omnia practica*, Paris, J. Dallin, 1664, pp. 510–11.
[85] In fact, *On the nature of man*, 14, Littré, vol. VI, p. 67.
[86] Lazare Rivière, *Observationes medicae et curationes insignes*, Paris, S. Piquet, 1646, pp. 15–16.
[87] Latin: *Meynenses*, probably not Mainz.
[88] Laurentius Scholz, *Consilia et Epistolae* in *Epistularum philosophicarum libri*, Hanover, Wechel, 1610.

The flesh of the woodland hedgehog can be substituted for the flesh of snakes. And it is not only good for elephantiasis cases, but also for sufferers from nephritis, cachexia, severe convulsions and those who suffer from dropsy, as Galen testifies in his chapter on Hedgehogs.[89]

Boerhaave, my much respected teacher, prescribed the following treatment for a lawyer aged 37 suffering since childhood from impetigo; see a description of the disease's history in Boerhaave's 'Consultations':[90]

"I have considered this disease and weighed in my mind how to make a trial of this method in the space of one and a half months. Firstly, every day, morning and evening, the affected skin areas should be thoroughly rubbed with warm dry cloths woven with rough, uncarded wool, which have been held above the fumes of heated sulphur so that they are saturated with vapour. Secondly, avoid fatty foods with a strong smell or aroma, smoked or dried with salt. Farinosa vegetables and green vegetables can be taken—very ripe fruits, also fresh white meat and freshwater fish. To drink: weak beer and a little French white wine is allowed. Thirdly, one hour before breakfast, lunch and dinner, 5 pills (A) should be swallowed followed immediately by drinking 5 oz of medicated liquor (B).

(A) Flowers of sulphur 3 scruples; Myrrh 1½ scruples; Rhubarb 1 scruple; Turpentine ½ scruple.
Make pills of 3 gr each.

(B) Freshly prepared meadow sorrel up to 1 peck; Grasses up to 2 pecks; Dandelions up to 1½ pecks; Sorrel root 3½ scruples. Boil with fresh milk for 2 hours then strain the liquid through a cloth.
Recently I have been giving 15 [oz] daily."

Sulphur water and salt waters from Moffat are of value in treating peeling and pimply skin as has been shown by considerable practical experience. George Sowerby, a butcher living in Carlisle, was completely cured of impetigo by using these remedies.

"There is another type of eruption but less frequent *which no evacuation at all helps to cure*. This condition occurs in other parts of the body, but especially on the chest and it settles in a fairly defined area, hardly protruding above the skin and looking like a more diffuse spot. Otherwise it appears scurfy and peeling with almost yellowish flakes. Whether the patient has maculae or full-blown impetigo, he is quite well in himself. When they are going away it often happens that he feels a little unwell and passes urine which is rather reddish and turbid, tinged with yellow. In the same way the patient can be improved by the treatment, keeping rigidly to the stated medicines after the general evacuation, and the same regime in severe itching and then not forgetting to allow the use of wines and easily digested meats, although refrigerants are more of a hindrance than a help. And so this worst type of eruption can be cured, although it sometimes yields only to vitriolated waters taken over a long period of time." Sydenham, p. 281.[91]

[89] Galen, *Opera omnia*, ed. C. G. Kühn, 20 vols in 22, Hildesheim, Georg Olms, 1964–65, vol. XII, p. 321.
[90] Hermann Boerhaave, *Consultationes medicae*, London, J. Nourse, 1744, pp. 102–3.
[91] Thomas Sydenham, *Opera universa*, Leiden, J. Kerchem, 1726.

After careful consideration of all this information I have decided to apply the following method of treatment.

May 1st, 1738

Matthew Rotchford's son.[92]

Venesection—about 8 oz of blood from an arm vein. The following night he should take the pills on retiring, then next morning at daybreak, he should take eight spoonfuls of hot apozem every half hour.

> Pill Rufus 25 gr; Borax 5 gr; Peruvian balsam 1 drop; Make 6 pills.
> Glauber's salts 3 scruples; Sal martis 1 scruple; Root of black hellebore 1½ scruples; Root of iris 1½ scruples; Liquorice root 3 scruples; Small cardamom seeds 1 scruple.
> Boil in spring water as required to 1 pt and in between the medicines he should drink copious draughts of milk stout.

May 4th

> Elderflower ointment 3 oz; Liquid tar 1 oz; Peruvian balsam 1 scruple. Stir together until liquified then apply to the affected parts every night on retiring.
> Sal martis 3 scruples; Black hellebore 1 scruple; Camphor ½ scruple; Extract of gentian ½ scruple; Copaiba balsam as required.
> Form into a mass for making pills, and make 10 pills, each of a single drachm. Two to be taken every morning at 6, 7 and 8 o'clock, followed by a large draught of posset.

By the second or third change of ointment, the peeling skin cleared up. The skin underlying it looked very fragile and red. He took the pills and as a result no noticeable change was observed except that he passed large amounts of urine. The course of pills was repeated.

May 25th. When by the fourth day all the ointment had been used up, thin, purplish flakes of skin began to break out again in the same place. I prescribed the following liniment:

> Apple ointment 2½ oz; Copaiba balsam 1 oz.
> Make a liniment with a very little, then rub on the affected areas every night on retiring.

October 18th, 1738

68 Mrs. William Gilpin,[93] a woman of frail physique, about 25, who suffered almost continually from chlorosis while single, but having been married for two years she enjoyed better health and she has given birth to a healthy, full-term boy. However, for the last two winters she has been covered in a rash, the same as I described in the case of the barber, but it appears mostly on her arms, especially around the elbows. At first the spots are small and not at all conspicuous. They become daily bigger and bigger and then peel in bran-like

[92] Matthew Rotchford must have been a valued and wealthy member of Whitehaven society to have persuaded Brownrigg to undertake this detailed search of medical sources on behalf of his son. It also indicated the books which the doctor had access to, either in his own library or that of his patron, Sir James Lowther—see Appendix V for the list of medical books in the Flatt inventory of 1757 (Carlisle Record Office: D/Lons/L Miscellaneous).

[93] Wife of William Gilpin, the son of the Lowthers' steward (1693–1722) and a merchant of the town. He was the co-owner of the Sugarhouse by 1729, based on imports from the West Indies.

flakes, the underlying skin being tinged with red, but this quickly fades. The rash appears at about the autumnal equinox and clears up with the arrival of the swallows.

Apple ointment 1½ oz; Coaltar liquid ½ oz; Peruvian balsam 1 scruple; Oil of lavender as required, so as to achieve a pleasant smell. Make a liniment to be applied every night.
Pill Ruffus ½ scruple. 6 pills to be taken on retiring.
Cream of tartar 3 scruples; Sal martis 1 scruple. To be divided into 6 papers. One to be taken every half hour with one spoonful of Scarborough water, beginning at 7 a.m., and Scarborough water to be taken while working.

A cathartic was repeated in turn. The spots became much bigger and one appeared on her shoulder and several on her cheek, which had not been seen in that area previously; then severe itching started on her arms and her skin became red. On the 29th October I prescribed the following pills:

Best rhubarb root 50 gr; Black hellebore root ½ scruple; Crocus ½ scruple; Amber salts ½ scruple; Sal martis 1½ scruples.
Sufficient silvery turpentine to make a fairly firm dough. Make 12 pills of 1 scruple, three to be taken every night on retiring and at 7 a.m. and 11 a.m. Every morning 1 pt of Spa water should be drunk.

May 1745

69 Miss Milham, a single woman aged 23, who had suffered since early adolescence from flaking and scurf of the skin like Scabies. She was otherwise healthy. For this condition she had tried all kinds of remedies, but in vain, to wit: Wardrew water, water from Lough Neagh in Ireland, and Scarborough water. After using this last treatment practically the whole of her skin was covered in whitish scurf, nor did the skin flakes disappear after using the waters for three weeks continuously. She then improved for 5 or 6 years, indeed throughout this time she was not troubled by any skin blemishes, but her hands and arms were always red and on them were little hard, rough areas of skin which in several places tended to crack. Her face, too, was red and often shiny from using coaltar ointment, for she often used this and only rarely did spots appear on other parts, i.e., hands, arms and face. Indeed, when drying northerly and easterly winds were blowing, her hands and her whole skin were covered again with blemishes of a yellowish colour, discharging fluid. Then the flakes fell off in dry layers which, when they dropped off, left the skin underneath red and then new flakes formed and rose up above it. She was constipated and for 4 or 5 years her menstrual periods were infrequent with only scanty loss. During her periods she suffered from abdominal cramps and joint pains. I prescribed the following:

2nd May.

Powdered electuarium of myrrh 2½ scruples; Root of black hellebore, finely powdered 1 scruple; Sal martis 2½ scruples; Extract of gentian 1 scruple; A sweet proprietary elixir; Amber oil 20 drops; Common pure vinegar 20 drops. Make up pills of 5 gr and take 3 in the hour before breakfast, lunch and dinner, followed by 2 spoonfuls of the apozem.
Guaiacum bark 5½ oz; Red sandalwood bark ½ oz; Root of sorrel 3 oz; Root of sea holly ½ oz; Liquorice root 1½ oz; Vitriolated tartar 1 oz; Strong cinnamon water 3 oz.

[English]

OF THE CHIN-COUGH

From D^r. Burton's Treatise on the Non-Naturals published at York, 1738.[94]

Physicians have not taken sufficient notice of this Disease and the present method of treating it is so long and tedious, that as Willis says "Because it failed to change for years, or be overcome by remedies". This disease rarely affects Adults, nor yet Infants, but when it becomes epidemical & is caused by a great quantity of thick Phlegm obstructing in, & adhering to the Lungs and parts adjacent, and the Phlegm is caused by the Laxity of the Fibres, and the diet of Children; by which means they become most liable to this Distemper.

The curative Indications are first to attenuate and dissolve the Phlegm; secondly to corroborate or strengthen the Fibres, to prevent any other viscidity. This viscid Humour is not only to be attenuated, but also evacuated. But purging would destroy one of the curative Indications, nay if the Patient when almost recovered, he would be in danger of a relapse, and the Author observed in two children, it is in many things like an intermitting fever as we shall also see, it has also been cur'd by Frights as well as the Ague as Willis tells us "How by a sudden fright children would be cured of the convulsive coughs".

As this Humour, therefore can't so safely be carried off by Stool, and by Vomiting it can't; we then have no other way but by Urine, which may safely be done; & how beneficial Diuretics are in many Disorders of the Lungs no Physician is ignorant.

He never bleeds, unless to gain time when there is Danger of a Convulsion, if the main passages (as it mostly happens) abound with Phlegm, then he gives a little Honey & Squills: or like and detersive purges, otherwise if he thinks the Medicine can get freely into the Lactials he neither Vomits, nor purges. For the first Intention of Cure he used Millepedes with the Testaceous powders; being administered for two or three days as he saw Occasion; which did not only cut & dislodge the Phlegm, but also carried a great deal of it off by Urine. He then administered the Peruvian Bark which Remedy is adapted, to answer both the Indications of Cures, for both by the Smallness, Solidity, & Irregularities of its Parts, as soon as it mixes with the Blood it cant but give it a greater Momentum, & increase the Impulses of its parts one against another, upon which Account a great many Cohesions will be broke, & other parts prevented from running into such close contacts as occasion those Cohesions. The other Intention will be answered by its corrugating the Fibres, by which means the ailment, & Humours will be better digested. This method I communicated to the late Dr. Woodhouse who found it to answer his Expectations. Thro the whole year 1730 the weather was moist & rainy but the year 1731 was exceeding dry & the Drought was so universal as is scarce to be paralleld in the Memory of Man. About the 24 of Decemb: 1731 it suddenly became a hard Frost, & so continued till the 29th & then as suddenly broke into a warm Thaw. It frose and thaw'd by Intervalls thro the whole month of January. In the Beginning of Feb: the frost quite ended but the weather remained cold and dry with northerly Winds till about the Middle of April, then some rain fell and the Winds were Easterly & Southerly till the beginning of May.

[94] John Burton, *A treatise on the non-naturals*, York, A. Staples & J. Hildyard, 1738, pp. 345–67.

About the Middle of January 1731:2, the Chin-Cough began to be very Epidemical & was more or less fatal as the Weather altered.

The Method above mentioned being followed in that Season by nineteen Children, 17 of em' recovr'd in so small a time as to show they were cured by the Medicine, & not by any Change in the Temperature of the Air.

One of those who did not live two days after I was sent for, & the other had several Convulsive Fitts before I was sent for. Upon a looseness coming, two of the Children who had recovered relapsed. During this Epidemical Season Agues were stirring, and the Sick had a troublesome Cough. In Octob: & Novemb: 1735 he cured more by the same Method. He has since used the following Medicines, by which he has cured the Disease very soon, sometimes in five or six days.

> Gentle purgative powders: Camphor 1 scruple; Extract of Peruvian bark 3 scruples. Mix together.
> If the symptoms appear again take 8 or 9 grains every 3 or 4 hours & a spoonful, occasionally or as well as the correct juleps in which Copaiba balsam should be dissolved.
> Drink the emulsion copiously as a common drink.

This method is not proper in such Chin Coughs as proceed from a thin sharp Rheum but I believe in that from a tough Viscid Phlegm it will scarce even fail, at least it has not fail'd yet.

For the Chin Cough Boerhaave prescribed phlebotomy, vomitory, cathartics repeatedly and bleeding. I well remember seeing this prescription in Mr. Garnière's chemist's shop in London.

[Latin]

CONVULSIVE COUGHING (I.E. THE CHIN-COUGH)

For the Rev. Dr. Ashley's two daughters, the elder being 8 years old and the younger 6, both suffering from convulsive coughing. After using leeches to extract blood, I prescribed the following on 23rd November 1741:

> Electuary of Peruvian bark 1 oz; Root of elecampane 1½ scruples; Wormwood ½ oz. Boil for half an hour in spring water and make up 1 pt, adding at the end:
> Gum arabic 1½ scruples; Liquorice root 2½ scruples; Aniseed seeds ½ scruple. Strain and add Tincture of Saffron 1 scruple.
> Make into an apozem.

The elder girl should take about 1 oz and the younger 6 scruples every 3 hours with the following drops:

> Tincture of cantharides ½ oz.

The elder to take 8 drops and the younger 6 drops in single doses, with the above decoction.

But it was in vain.[95]

[95] Later faint addition.

NOTES ON HAEMORRHOIDS

1. Which vessels cause the bleeding.

   Vesalius, in his book on the Fabric of the human body (Vol. 5, Chapter 15)[96] reminds us of a man who used to suffer from bleeding from the veins surrounding the anus at fixed periods, just like women during their monthly periods. When he died from deep jaundice and a greatly hardened liver, it was noticed, when about to dissect and see whether the branches of the portal or caval vein had discharged this blood, that the branch of the portal vein at the distal end of the colon which runs the whole length of the rectum into the mesentery, was almost as thick as his thumb and swollen with blood (a).

   (a) In the same work, Vesalius (Book 3, Chapter 5)[97] says "Occasionally, in those suffering from haemorrhoids throughout the body as a whole, I have seen a yellowish fluid regurgitate towards the branches of the vena cava which are in the region of the perineum". This is very similar to our own and I have noted it while I have been examining the true distribution of the portal system. This adds great force to my opinions, although I have not dissected any haemorrhoid cases with this reflux of blood for a long time, and in these cases the spleen was smaller and harder and the vein running along beneath the rectum was more than the thickness of the thumb. It was swollen with blood in the same way that I have seen in pregnant animals, the veins surrounding the uterus noticeably full and distended.

   From Bonet *Sept: Anat:* See Book 2, p. 277, observation 1.[98]

2. Bleeding sometimes occurs before puberty.

   I desire to note in passing, on the subject of haemorrhoids, a case that quite recently occurred in a boy aged 11, although Hippocrates' second book, *Coac: Prenot: Aph:* p. 512 states "Haemorrhoids do not exist before puberty, but appear in the late stages of adolescence, Aph: 30. Sect. 3".[99] It seems that this haemorrhoidal bleeding can be caused by worms. The boy's parents noticed these creatures around his anus and the bleeding followed a short time afterwards.

3. As I write, a girl of 9 has been sent to me for treatment suffering from haemorrhoids due to the same cause. Mollebranch. *De Varis.*[100]

4. Periodic bleeding haemorrhoids in men.

   I once knew a man who suffered from bleeding haemorrhoids every month and who is now over 80. Anton: Zimara, from Marcell: Donat: p. 411.[101]

[96] Vesalius, *De humani corporis fabrica*, Basle, J. Oporinus, 1543, p. 537.

[97] Ibid., p. 267.

[98] Théophile Bonet, *Sepulchretum sive anatomia practica ex cadaveribus morbo denatis*, Geneva, Cramer and Perachon, 1700.

[99] Littré, vol. IV, p. 501.

[100] Valentin Andreas Moellenbrock, *De varis seu arthritide vaga scorbutica tractatus*, Leipiz, G. Michaelis for J. Gross, 1672.

[101] Marcellus Donatus, *De historia medica*, Frankfurt, J. J. Porsius, 1613.

5. Just as women become obese because of their laxer fibres and experience discharges of blood with advantage to their health, so men also of this same type and physical structure, by reason of excess blood frequently produce blood from the haemorrhoidal veins. These vessels, if the plethora is reduced, shrink and discharge mucous lymph just like menstrual discharge from the uterus, and very occasionally it can happen that these men suffer from a white discharge from time to time, which is very like the discharge which often affects women. Woodhouse. Inaugural thesis. p. 11 of Hist:[102]

6. Sir Wilfred Lawson [of Isel Hall, Cockermouth] has told me that for thirty years or more he has suffered from periodic rectal bleeding and that before he passes the blood he feels severe colicky pain, and moreover that the bleeding was caused on the first occasion by using Tinct. Sacra on the advice of Dr. Radcliffe. Quite often before the onset of this bleeding he feels generalised arthritic pains which are relieved immediately by the passage of blood. Only once did he suffer from an extremely severe attack of joint pains which occurred after he had been free from the bleeding for two years. However, when the bleeding occurred, his kidney pains, which had troubled him severely at other times, were relieved, and almost every week he picked out two or three small stones passed during micturition. My observation.

   Query: Quantity and quality of discharged blood at each occasion? Intervals between bleeds? Did he himself suffer from the occasional headaches of which he spoke?

7. In some cases this passage of blood takes place through haemorrhoids, as Amat: Lusitanus, Book 5.32, and Bartholomeus' Chapter 5.33[103] noted that, in others, haemoptysis occurs from time to time, and in not a few, recurrent passage of bloodstained urine is to be seen. Indeed the same passage of blood occurs in women through plethora and it often benefits their health and if their usual cleansing discharge is suppressed, then they become ill, as Salmathus recalls: "If the occasional passage of blood-stained urine ceases, then a tremendous and powerful tightness of the chest and the greatest difficulty in breathing occur, and the patient may die of this within a few days". By the same token, if ulcers and eruptions, which for a long time have been wont to bleed suddenly dry up, they empty, causing considerable danger.

   Friend [*sic*]. *Emmenolog.:* Chapter 8.[104]

8. Lusitanus, Cur: 3, of the 5th Century, writes that Johannes Baptista Propola, at the age of forty-five, had copious bleeding from haemorrhoids each month, just as the menstrual flow affects women. If this was checked and did not flow in the usual way,

[102] J. Woodhouse, *Dissertatio de medicina instituenda et promovenda*, Leiden, 1700.

[103] Amatus Lusitanus, *Curationum medicinalium centuriae septem*, Barcelona, S. and J. Mathevat, 1628, p. 890. Bartolomeus reference not identified.

[104] J. Freind, *Emmenologia*, in *Opera omnia*, London, J. Wright, 1733, p. 86.

then he produced blood from his mouth without any cough or fever, in many reddish-yellow clots. He was cured when his haemorrhoids bled. From M. Donat: p. 411.[105]

9. Sometimes they take the place of menses in women. A certain woman who had her uterus surgically removed, when the time of her period was due, had a monthly flow from the nearby anus at the usual time and of the same colour. Having been restored to health, she lived for a long time afterwards without having to use any other treatment, and when this monthly flow through the anus was rather sluggish, the vein next to the malleolus was opened.

   Platerus: *Observations: Med:* Book 3.[106]

   A respectable married woman showing the symptoms of pregnancy and at the same time obstruction of the anus, was meanwhile attacked by very severe pain in the anal region. I have determined the cause of her obstruction of the haemorrhoidal veins. Horstius: p. 255. T.2.[107]

10. Throughout the literature there are many references to women who, when their menstrual flows ceased, were improved in health by passing blood at the due times, but from haemorrhoids.

    Sennert: *Prax:* Book 3[108] and Bonet: *Med: Sept:* 36[109] from Friend [*sic*]: *Emmenolog.*[110]

11. Also in pregnant women.

    I too have noted that haemorrhoids can bleed to good effect in pregnant women—e.g., in two noblewomen who were four months pregnant, a full time delivery followed, which proceeded in a completely normal manner.

    Hollerus [*sic*] in *Praxis.*[111]

12. They cure many illnesses.

    Equally Lusitanus writes: Cent: 2: Case 13[112]—that Angelus de Prato used to suffer from copious bleeding from haemorrhoids. When he tried many cures they stopped and it came about that in spring there were emissions of blood from his mouth. When the haemorrhoids were incised, he lived unharmed by this bringing up of blood.

    Also from Donatus.

12.b Bleeding haemorrhoids.

I have seen a divine, incredible and miraculous treatment, followed by such amazing results that unlearned people believed it to be a miracle. Now I have

[105] Donatus, *De historia medica*, 1613.
[106] Felix Plater, *Observationes*, Basel, L. König, 1641, bk 3, pp. 718–19.
[107] Horst, *Opera medica*, 1661, vol. 2, p. 255.
[108] Daniel Sennert, *Practicae medicinae liber primus (—sextus)*, Paris, 1633.
[109] Théophile Bonet, *Medicina septentrionalis*, bk 3, pp. 81–9.
[110] Freind, *Emmenolog.*, in *Opera omnia*, 1733, p. 103.
[111] Hollerius, *De morbis internis*, in *Opera omnia*, 1664, p. 430.
[112] Amatus Lusitanus, *Curationum medicinalium centuriae septem*, 1628, p. 280.

observed such events in the case of a famous British physician who was suffering from mania. I forbade him to be bound, but instead I ordered him to take aloes every hour. After 12 hours he complained of pain around the anus and at the same moment there was a brisk discharge of blood. Immediately he regained his sanity. This discharge from the internal arteries is most healthgiving. Enemas may be administered first, and if that is not sufficient then suppositories made from aloes should be used. If this is still not enough the parts should be bathed with warm milk and horse leeches applied. The patient should then be placed on a commode with some hot water and the blood can be heard trickling forth and so can be disposed of at will.

Boerhaave in *Praelectionib: privatis:* Aph: 702 on Delirium.[113]

13. I have noted when horse leeches are applied to external haemorrhoids about two measures of material similar to frogspawn have flowed forth and the patient has been freed from long-standing troubles, passing wind, persistent pain and other symptoms. Sorbait. *Op*. p. 420.[114]

14. I have also known quite a few cases where the discharge of blood from haemorrhoids has been caused by scurvy, and several women who have recovered their health when their menses flowed at short intervals.
Bald: Ronsseus. On Scurvy.[115]

15. Mr. Lawson has told me that an occasional discharge from his haemorrhoids (see above, section 6), cured him of livid patches on his sides, and other serious symptoms of scurvy. Our observation.

16. Ambroise Paré the surgeon told me of a nobleman admitted to his hospital, and invited me to a consultation, because when the man suffered from severe renal colic he passed blood, pus and thick mucus. Having indicated the nature of his treatment because he had haemorrhoidal swellings and because the pain did not respond to other remedies, I immediately ordered the haemorrhoids to be incised, as a result of which the pain settled down with amazing speed. Hollerus [*sic*].[116]

17. Mrs. Fisher, a widow aged 40, had been suffering for two days from severe back pains, shaking fits, and trembling of the muscles in her back, and severe pains in the uterus all at the same time. There was no evidence of fever, vomiting, or signs of the stone;* however, when her external haemorrhoids swelled up she was free from all her pain for a short time. Our observation. August 1738.
*The symptoms were relieved by using manna enemas and other laxative treatments and anodynes. Before this treatment this lady had been greatly grieved

[113] Boerhaave, *Aphorismi*, 1715, p. 140.
[114] Paul de Sorbait, *Universa medicina*, Nuremberg, J. and F. Endter, 1672.
[115] Balduinus Ronsseus, *De magnis Hippocratis lienibus . . . seu . . . scorbuto commentarius*, in D. Sennertus, *De scorbuto*, Frankfort & Wittenberg, Hiers of T. Marius, & E. Schumacher, 1654.
[116] Hollerius, *Opera omnia*, p. 430.

both by the death of her husband and also because her monthly periods had not appeared for a long time. Afterwards some spots appeared on her skin and spread all over her body, as happens frequently to those with irregular periods.

18. A patient in his forties had been much troubled by a hard prominent tumour in the middle of his chest for a long time, and having been treated by useless remedies first internally and then externally for nine months, he was in despair concerning his health. Suddenly a discharge occurred and at once the aforesaid chest swelling disappeared, to his astonishment, and the patient recovered. Riverius or Horstius.

19. Side effects of suppression of haemorrhoids.

    Hippocrates Book 3: *Epid:*[117] tells the story of Alcippus who, having haemorrhoids, suppressed the symptoms by means of treatment and then, being cured, became insane. From Donatus.

20. I can confirm that the suppression of haemorrhoids, to whom formerly it was second nature to have bleeding almost every month, was to me an especial cause of illness (indeed of very severe and sudden arthritic pain in a man previously free from this disease). Petrus Monavius in Scholzii: *Epist*: p. 421.[118]

21. A certain patient was often seized by redness and swelling of his fingers. Though curing his haemorrhoids by means of useless remedies prolonged the problem, as soon as his haemorrhoids bled his symptoms vanished next day. Riverius or Horstius.

22. Excessive haemorrhoidal bleeding.

    A respected married lady aged about forty had been suffering from excessive bleeding from external haemorrhoids for eight months, with the result that she had become extremely cachectic and tending to dropsy, with complete muscular weakness so that she could hardly walk. She had a yellowish appearance of her face and whole body. At length the bleeding was completely cured by the appropriate treatment; however, after a month she felt burning pain in her upper abdomen and suffered from restless nights. It was easy to assume this was caused by the retention of the blood which had previously been discharged from her haemorrhoids, and which her nature could not control properly, so accustomed was it to these evacuations especially when her menstruation had stopped for some years. So I prescribed venesection, with the beneficial result that her symptoms were relieved. Riverius: *Obs*: p. 546.[119]

[117] Littré, vol. V, p. 197.

[118] Scholz, *Consilia et Epistolae*, 1610.

[119] Lazare Rivière, *Observationes*, in either *Opera medica universa*, Lyons, J. Hugueton, 1679, or the later edition also published in Lyons by Anisson and J. Posuel in 1698.

23. I recall the example of a married woman with very severe and longstanding haemorrhoidal bleeding requiring diligent and energetic treatment. I saw her physically exhausted and quite demoralised, threatened with the considerable risk of slowing down the flow of blood. Indeed from the first day of the cure she was much burdened by the consequences, for she swelled up around the precordial region and began to develop oedema. I was called in on the sixth day, and opened up the closed-up veins to restart the flow, but I could not check them safely and heavily before making sure about slight bodily evacuations and other strengthening means for that vital organ, the liver. Verzascha: *Obs*: p. 90.[120] from Solenander: *Cons*: 2: Sect: 4.[121]

24. Daniel Horstius in *Op*. Tom. iii. p. 261[122] writes of his father James who died from excessive bleeding haemorrhoids when all remedies proved vain.

25. Haemorrhoids can cure gout.
Mr. Cornelius Zuyt, President of Holland, when he was suffering from arthritis, developed bleeding from his haemorrhoids which he had for a long time, and I told him straight away that he would be freed from all joint pains, nor did my opinion fail me, since they are also a remedy for kidney troubles. Forestus: *Obs*: 4. Book 23.

26. Quartan fever, cured by haemorrhoids.
John Heuterus, a respected citizen, was cured of a quartan fever and developed internal haemorrhoids near to the condylomata causing very severe pains, so that he spent all night awake and was very miserable because of a thick discharge of black bile. After being much troubled for a long time by this illness he was eventually cured by Forestus and a surgeon. See the case history described by Forestus: *Obs*: 7. Book 23.

27. Haematuria caused by suppression of haemorrhoidal bleeding.
A man who had long suffered from haemorrhoids and was controlling the bleeding himself, while consuming large quantities of food and wine and living a life of idleness, developed haematuria from time to time, the blood piling up in large quantities and finding its way round by another route, the haemorrhoids being held in check as often happened. Forestus. *Obs*: 9. Book 24.[123]

28. Melancholy due to suppression of haemorrhoidal bleeding and cured by restarting the flow.
A man over 30, hairy and of a very high colour, with frail constitution, was occasionally low in spirits because of various cares, and depressed at times. His haemorrhoids usually bled, but when the flow was checked he was seized by

[120] Bernhard Verzascha, *Observationum medicarum centuria*, Basle, J. J. Decker for H. Wetstenius, 1677.
[121] Reinert Solenander, *Consilia medicinalia*, Frankfurt, Heirs of Wechel, C. Marnius, & J. Aubrius, 1596, pp. 310–12.
[122] In fact this appears in vol. ii. The author is Gregor Horst, and the dead man was his uncle.
[123] Petrus Forestus, *Observationes et curationes medicinales*, Leiden, F. Raphelengius, 1596, pp. 44–5.

melancholy. When I went to see him I noticed he had a look of vague empty thoughts on his face. I noticed that the offending humour was not quite bad, only rodent, and was harmful only through the abundance of the fluid. He felt great heaviness of the body, had no perception of feeling, his face was much ruddier than before and his veins were greatly swollen and distended. When his haemorrhoidal bleeding was restarted by the usual method, he became quite sane again. See the whole case history related at length by Forestus. *Obs*: 14. Book 15.

29. *Obs*: 7. Book 15[124] also tells of a famous theologian and exceptionally gifted preacher who was completely cured of melancholy by encouraging his haemorrhoids to bleed.

30. Rondelet's wife died in the space of a few days from infected haemorrhoids which she wanted to hide from her husband. When the affected area was examined, the exterior part of the central area was found to be gangrenous. Bonet: *Sept*: *Anat*: Tome 2. p. 278. Obs: 2 from Joubert in the life of Rondelet.[125]

31. The two spleens of a young man were beautifully formed, each with its own blood supply from arteries and veins, and the largest haemorrhoidal veins came forth from the middle of the spleen. Although he was seen to be of the melancholic humour, he never throughout his whole life assumed a sad face. He was the darling of Jove, not Saturn. Same source. Obs: 3 from Cabrollius. *Obs: Anatom*: 15.[126]

32. Signor Marchetti stated that the external haemorrhoidal veins do not arise from the vena cava, but are branches of the portal vein and that the smallest twigs perforate the skin itself and finally end in tiny swellings beneath the cuticle. Leeches are applied to them. Sometimes the haemorrhoidal vein arises from the splenic branch, at other times from the mesenteric branch, but most frequently from a division of the portal vein. This vein distributes its branches to the entire small intestine.

Dr. Ray in *Philosophical Transactions*, Vol. 2, Part 2, p. 5,[127] in his account of Marchetti's Courses of Anatomy at Padua, thought this opinion somewhat improbable.

33. A white discharge from haemorrhoids.

A man aged 49, a chronic hypochondriac, developed severe haemorrhoids after purging and sought to have them lanced. When they were incised, out came material just like frogspawn, up to 10 fluid oz, with however some loss of strength, and he

[124] In 28 and 29 Brownrigg added the book references later, and wrongly; they should be: Forestus, *Observationes medicinales*, Antwerp, R. Plantin, 1602, Obs. 14, bk 10, pp. 337–8; Obs. 12, bk 10, pp. 326–8.

[125] Bonet, *Sepulchretum sive anatomia practica*, 1770; the Joubert reference has not been identified.

[126] Barthélemy Cabrol, *Alphabet anatomie*, Tournon, C. Michel and G. Linocier, 1594, pp. 94–5.

[127] *The Philosophical Transactions from the year 1700 to 1720*, Abridg'd, Part II, London, B. Motte, 1721, vol. 25, no. 307, 1706, p. 2289.

recovered from that very moment. Thus he was freed from this longstanding complaint and from a multitude of other troubles. *Ephemerid: German:* Year 1. Obs: 75.[128]

34. Very scanty haemorrhoidal bleeding each month in a male patient.
I heard of a waller, now dead, who from the age of 20 until he was 60, suffered from monthly bleeding from haemorrhoids, just like the menstruation of a young girl, and which recurred on a regular basis. If the bleeding stopped he was affected by the same symptoms as those of retained menstrual products or of a very scanty flow, and whether the flow came forth or stopped, by the same remedies as those of a young girl. *Ephemerid: German:* Year 2. Obs: 192.[129]

35. On excessive bleeding of haemorrhoids in an old woman.
See Observat: D. Georgii Wolfg. Wedelin in *Ephemerid: German:* Year 3. Obs 22: p. 39.

36. On monthly bleeding from the anus.
See Obs. by the same author in the same year. Obs: 24, p. 41.[130]

37. On an amulet of sure efficacity, that is the Root of Telephus.
See Observations of the same author in *Ephemerid: German:* Year 2. Obs: 194.[131]

38. On the arbitrary suppression of haemorrhoidal bleeding by the sole use of aromatic resins.
Ephemerid: German: Year 3. Obs: 226, p. 411.

39. On the method of suppressing haemorrhoids.
Gabriel von Hund, Governor of Grotkau [Silesia], had been afflicted for a long time by bleeding from haemorrhoids and was able to obtain relief from no one. Dr. Sebizius cured him with ointment made from tobacco, so that the flow was reduced, but quartan fever and scurvy followed and he died. *Ephemerid: German:* Year 3. Obs: 331, p. 543.

[Inserted note pasted in the Casebook.]

Mrs. Whitlock.

An electuary of Ammoniac gum 3 scruples; Electuary of myrrh 2 scruples; Camphor ½ scruple; Best rhubarb ½ scruple; Gentian extract 1 scruple; Liquorice 2 scruples; Common pure turpentine.
Make up a pill of ½ scruple for a headache.
Take one at dawn and at night for two whole months.

[128] *Miscellanea curiosa medico-physica academiae naturae curiosorum*, Leipzig, 1670, p. 157.
[129] Ibid., 1671, p. 294.
[130] Ibid., 1672.
[131] Ibid., 1671, p. 296.

Take 6 warm spoonfuls of this decoction.
Root of fresh burberry 2 oz; Twitchgrass 1 ½ oz; Guaiacum 3 scruples; Red sandalwood 3 scruples; Currants 1 oz; Vitriolated tartar 1 scruple. Boil for half an hour in spring water to make up 2 pts, and add when boiling:
Liquorice root 1 oz; Dried sea holly 1 oz; Roses 1 oz; Sassafras bark 1 oz. Strain, and add:
Strong cinnamon water 2 oz; Tincture of saffron 1 scruple.

[Inserted note pasted in the Casebook. This is a list of books, obviously used by Brownrigg when assembling his thoughts on haemorrhoids. It has been transcribed exactly as he set it down; some of the works can be found in Appendix V.]

Terra Mot 346 Etmuller.
Haemorrhoids ii 172+Various items 170+with
Morb. Hypochond examine iii 170+.
Tractus Haemorrhoid ii 172+
De Haemorrhoid Casus—iii 1135
" " Inflamationes tollere ii 387+
" " How to reveal them ii 167+iii 139.
Laco—Observationes iii 726—iii 735
Caec. Dolentib—Consultation—iii 164.
+Caeca a partu—ii 104–
+Tumour in gravid—ii 1008
—Riverii Ob.
318 Fluxus Hepatic 486–502
Fluxus Haemorrhoid immodicus per sedatus 570–576 cohabitus.

In feb Pestilent. (Ob G. Apertio Artific) 757–
In Calculo renum 349.
Ob gen.
+In Uteri Schirro 388. In Ischiade 457
In Tenesmo 306.
Haemorrhoid. Dolor. (quomodo superaedo. 280)
45. sanatus.
De Haemorrhoidib. 312 ch. sequentib. tractat 313. Casus Curationis
Haemorrhoid (blotted out).
Unde Febre pestilentiali moriebatur ex A. Massaria.
314. Inflationes tumores & curae praecedent. ab Haemorrhoid intempestive suppresis ex Solenander.
315. Haemorrohoid; a Uteris Procedentia e Amato Lusitano.
Inflam. et Ulcere. Ani, Piso pag 31 de Tenesmo p. 27.

[The following two lines are written upside down:]

Etmuller De fluxu Hepatico—Tom ii p 170.
De Haemorrhoidib.—Tom ii p 142.

[Small pages inserted in the Casebook.]

A truly remarkable case. A desperately serious illness with very dangerous cachexia, cured by haemorrhoids.

Thomas Iredale, a hard working hatter, aged about 46, a robust, hard working man of good constitution, although a hard beer drinker.

Had he any other illnesses?

Had his haemorrhoids bled previously?

Did he suffer from a cough every winter?

About the beginning of November 1748 he began to suffer from marked abdominal distension and swelling of the hypochondrium. At the same time he was seriously troubled by a cough and brought up large amounts of thin frothy sputum. He almost lost his appetite for food and also refused all drinks. Gradually his skin became yellowish in colour, his faeces became hard and lumpy, while his urine turned red, thick and frothy—signs of deterioration in his condition—with gradual loss of strength, so that he was reduced to a state of marked debility.

Possibly his illness was aggravated by a long sharp spell of frost which was raging that year, for he became worse, so that when I first saw him about February 8th he was reduced to a state of gross weakness and wasting. Together with these recent symptoms, there now developed enormous leucophlegmatic swellings of the legs, insatiable thirst, persistent nausea and frequent vomiting of everything he swallowed. He also had considerable fever with a weak, rapid pulse and in addition his cough grew much worse so that he was spending the whole of every night without sleep. The hypochondrial swelling increased so that he complained bitterly of severe pain. Having taken careful note of all these factors, I considered the patient's complaints to be quite justified, especially as his stomach could scarcely take the laxative apozem and the leaves of other plants with saffron which I prescribed. This was jaundice due to a large infarction of the liver. I would like to ask everyone if this is a hopeless case, but when after one or two days I noticed a considerable amount of frank blood being passed after he had moved his bowels, there was a ray of hope for his recovery.

And so, I decided to promote this bleeding from his internal haemorrhoids with all vigour, and to this end I prescribed the following pills—Pill Ruffi. This caused diarrhoea and tenesmus. As he had vomited almost all the pills given to him, I prescribed the treatment again, but this time as suppositories composed of 1 oz honey, 1 scruple salt and 2 scruples of aloes. At last his stomach settled a little, and then I prescribed the pills once more, with the result that he passed several stools with a considerable amount of blood and other material which was thick, streaked with blood and clotted. This passage of blood continued for two weeks, then I prescribed a julep. During this time the swelling, pain, and hypochondrial distention gradually cleared up. The thirst, fever and cough which had been resistant to treatment until then practically ceased, his stomach became able to take and digest light meals satisfactorily, he passed very satisfactorily quantities of urine, and his pale stools returned to the normal colour. Meanwhile the dropsical swelling of his legs disappeared on treatment with apozems and woods, and now being quite free from his illness he began working at his occupation in his lightest garments, as is the custom among these men.

March 4th. From that time till the present he has remained in perfect health except when he indulged in excessive amounts of beer.

Question—has he had other attacks in the past, or was he very fit from childhood onwards?

Had he had previous haemorrhoidal bleeding?

Fresh blood was discharged from his haemorrhoids for two weeks. On February 8th and during the next few days I prescribed for him, this being the first time I had seen him:[132]

Powdered guiaicum 2 oz; Powdered sandalwood 3 oz; Root of elecampane 1 oz; Root of iris 1 oz; Crushed raisins 1½ oz; Tartar salt 2 scruples.
Boil in a closed vessel with spring water to make up 2 pts. After straining add:
Root of sea holly 6 scruples; Liquorice root 6 scruples; Sandalwood bark 1 oz.
Allow the decoction to cool; strain and add: Cinnamon water 1½ oz.
Take 5 spoonfuls 4 times a day with the following electuary: Powdered crabs eyes 1½ scruples; Nitre 6 scruples; Wormwood 15 gr; Powdered olibanum 1 scruple; Pure common turpentine 2 scruples; Rose hip syrup 1½ oz.
Pill Ruffus.
Nitre salt.
Honey 1 drachm; Sal martis 1 scruple; Aloes 1 scruple.
Make a suppository. Feb 10. Strong cinnamon water 3½ oz; Alex water 3½ oz; Strong cinnamon 6 scruples; Paeony 6 scruples; Tincture of saffron 1½ scruples; Lavender spirit 1½ scruples; Sweet syrup of nitre ½ scruple; Sugar.
Make a julep and take 2 spoonfuls every 4th hour.

[Note inserted in the Casebook.]

My own case history when suffering from haemorrhoids.[133]

For a long time I have been suffering from pains in the legs and throughout my whole body in the mornings. My urine was straw-coloured but produced no sediment. I took myrrh for a long time and this caused heating of my body and constipation.

July 9th—Priapism all day.

July 10th (1st day of illness). In the morning, after passing a motion, I first of all felt a small external haemorrhoid at one side of the anus. At almost the same moment I felt tremendous heat throughout my body with flushing of my face and slight headache. My nostrils felt blocked so that I could hardly breathe, just as in catarrh. I ate a light lunch; however in the afternoon the feelings of heat and flushing were extremely troublesome. In the evening there was internal pain from the haemorrhoid. At bedtime I took Pill Ruffus, but the pain was worse during the night.

July 11th (2nd day of illness). Morning—in great pain. I took 3 scruples of cream of tartar with tartarised whey. I passed seven stools in the day. I had thirst, and severe pain in the haemorrhoid which was not throbbing but was tense and causing pain which really

[132] This man was a hard beer drinker. He had abdominal distenstion, poor appetite, nausea and some jaundice, in addition to bleeding haemorrhoids, all of which suggests liver disease, complicating his alcoholism.

[133] This hastily written set of observations on his own case may account for the lengthy investigation of the works on haemorrhoids. It must perhaps be assumed that Brownrigg carried out his own surgery as there is no mention of his consulting a colleague, perhaps trusting more to his own aseptic techniques than those of others. He must have been a dedicated doctor to ride 6 miles (possibly to a patient) on horseback only 8 days after carrying out the operation, and while the incisions were still discharging. No date is indicated for this episode of Brownrigg's indisposition, a secondarily infected thrombosis in an external or prolapsed pile.

made me suffer with strangury. It was aggravated by coughing or any other exertion. Especially after being at stool, three haemorrhoids like grapes appeared at one side of the anus and were very tense and they discharged a foul thick fluid with a pungent smell like a fish called Ling. Evening—Terrible pain. I could neither sit down nor walk about without severely aggravating the pain and there was pain in my back too. One haemorrhoid was incised with a lancet and from the open wound there came forth hard thick clots of blood the size of a kidney bean. Thereafter the blood flowed out slowly. At night—the pain was worse, I had a fever, I was restless and my temples were throbbing.

July 12th. Morning—2 other haemorrhoids were incised and discharged thick clotted blood at first. From all of them, the blood was hard, thick and dark but friable and it flowed all the time, in small quantities but continually. The pain was somewhat relieved and I frequently applied linen cloths soaked in water, with which I washed the affected part and bathed it. At night the pain grew worse and my temples throbbed.

July 13th. When the blood had trickled from the incisions after the haemorrhoids had been lanced, they became flaccid and subsided. Pain now a little better. Bowels opened with tartarised whey.

July 14th. Still some bleeding but more serous. Pain much improved so that I could sit fairly comfortably at stool.

July 15th. Bleeding more serous and in smaller amounts, but with a more offensive odour. The anal cleft was very sore due to the continual dampness and rubbing of the affected area, and the sharp pain from this was now worse than from the haemorrhoids themselves.

July 16th, 17th, 18th, 19th and 20th. The fluid discharge is now gradually becoming more viscous and more sticky. It is yellow and less offensive.

July 19th. I rode 6 miles on horseback after sitting at stool. Blood still discharging from the external haemorrhoids.

July 24th. There still remains one small haemorrhoid, rather damp with mucus, but it is small and painless. The rest have almost completely gone. Appetite better than before the attack, colour much better, urine is straw-coloured but without sediment. Health good.

DISSERTATION ON HAEMORRHOIDS

What is Haemorrhois? The word haemorrhois properly means a bloodstained discharge from the haemorrhoidal veins and in that sense was first accepted by the ancient authors.

> According to Forestus, Book 23. Ob. 3.[134] "Haemorrhoids are nothing other than varicose veins in the anus". Bonet. *Anat. Pract.* Folio 2. p. 278. from Waleus.[135]

Some writers have used the word in a wider sense so that they have also understood the term to mean haemorrhoidal swelling around the vessels, whether with or without the discharge of blood or other fluids. So, many different terms have been proposed for haemorrhoids, depending on their size and appearance. They are described as being like little grapes, blackberries, warts or cysts and the affected area can be external or internal.

[134] Forestus, *Observationes et curationes*, 1596.

[135] Bonet, *Sepulchretum sive anatomia practica*, 1700. The reference is probably to Johannes Walaeus' *Epistuale duae de motu chyli et sanguinis*, which had various printings.

According to the symptoms, they may be painful or inflamed; moreover, those which bleed or are easily seen are called "open" while those which lie unseen inside and do not bleed at all are called "hidden".

> Others called these haemorrhoids "open" when they discharge blood and "hidden" when they are sited high up, and again they differentiate between "effluent" and "sealed" haemorrhoids. "It is known that in widows, haemorrhoids bleed satisfactorily in place of the menses". Forestus.
>
> "Haemorrhoids are wont to appear in some cases at intervals; in some every five years, and in others once every year or more often as in those who lose a lot of blood. There are moreover, haemorrhoids which bleed at regular intervals, as in elderly widows and in others whose menses have ceased". Id. Book 23. Obs. 5.

To whom is this illness most familiar? Those people who are often affected by haemorrhoids are of the melancholy temperament, and those who live in hot regions are more familiar with it than those in cold areas. According to the testimony of Hippocrates they do not bleed before puberty, but may (if we can trust the old writers) sometimes affect rare cases otherwise. Between the ages of 21 and 35 they occur at times, but rarely. In adult males from the age of 35 to 49, also in those approaching old age they most often begin to bleed. In women, after the age of 49. Men exhibit regular haemorrhoidal bleeding similar to the menses of women. Also pregnant women who are obese, throughout the three or four months after conception have beneficial relief from extra blood flowing from the haemorrhoidal vessels.

Causes of Haemorrhoids. The following causes of haemorrhoids are enumerated throughout the writings of ancient authors:

(a) Plethora, which often occurs in maimed limbs or in those who indulge in excessive eating or to those who have given up activities which they formerly practised. For instance, those who have omitted to take their usual exercise, or whose usual bleeding has stopped, or whose habit has been to compress the vessels and accelerate the process. In these cases haemorrhoids arise and then they often produce suppression of the menses in turn.

> On the other hand, Aristotle mentions women in whom the menses responded well and did not form varicose bleeding or haemorrhoidal veins.

(b) Bad digestion, arising from a strong strain of melancholy humour, which often affects those who use thick foods, hard to digest, who wear themselves out with strenuous drinking bouts or who are weighed down all day with cares and sadness or live a sedentary life or, finally, those who apply themselves too earnestly to their studies, especially at night.

(c) Whatever prevents the blood from returning freely from the haemorrhoidal veins to the heart, such as obstructions of the liver and colon. To be avoided are: violent exertion in labour and in defaecation, hardened faeces in the bowel, bladder stones, procidentia* of the uterus or anus.

*Riverius gives an example in Book 10. *Prax*. Ch. 11. From Lusitanus *Cur*. 19. Cen. 2.[136]

[136] Lazare Rivière, *Praxis medica* in *Opera medica universa*, Lyons, J. Hugueton, 1679, p. 315; the reference to Amatus Lusitanus has not been identified.

Other inflammations or tumours in the neighbourhood of the anus, all of which compress the haemorrhoidal veins.

(d) Powerful irritants and stimulants which are taken internally or applied externally in large quantities. The aloes cure has the special power to cause weakness of these veins and the following also possess the property: saffron; root or juice of cyclamen; juice of squills; beef gall; the seed of wild grape, etc., administered in the form of an enema or suppository. In addition it is possible to enumerate other irritants and erosive substances, either mechanical or caused by friction, i.e. harsh anastomatics, horseriding and worms.

(e) Weakness of the haemorrhoidal vessels, whence arises in some the disease as a result of the bodily construction they were born with. This weakness is often produced also by artificial means; by the use of laxatives in the form of vapour; fomenting; poultices and the administration of clysters. "In the elderly long afflicted by arthritis, when because of physical weakness there are irregular shaking attacks". These patients are often greatly troubled by pain in the vessels, as the great Sydenham has observed.

(f) Finally, fever can often be the cause of haemorrhoids.

Forestus mentions afflictions of spirit among the forementioned causes. V.L. fear, torment and afflictions of spirit.

DIAGNOSIS OF HAEMORRHOIDS

External haemorrhoids, whether bleeding or not, are easily diagnosed on sight. Internal haemorrhoids can be recognised by swelling or inflammation. If one of the aforementioned causes has already occurred; if the bowel is moved only with great difficulty due to swelling of the anus; if there has been constipation for many days; if suppositories and enemas can only be introduced with difficulty; if intense violent pain is present with the most dreadful stabbing sensation which is made much worse by compressing the anus and by passing a stool with great effort, and by tenesmus or a feeling of heaviness around the anal area and that the lower parts have been turned inside out by continual efforts as though all the abdominal organs were about to be expelled, or by strangury or inflammation of the nearby bladder.

If haemorrhoids are situated near the anal margin, then the prolapsed bowel is obvious to the observer, especially if the patient has been straining at stool and has previously bathed the area with warm water. The blood flowing through the anus can be diagnosed as coming from bleeding haemorrhoidal veins if the signs of swelling or inflammation appear at the same time, although often haemorrhoids bleed without any swelling or feeling of pain. They always bleed during attempts to move the bowels and most of all they pour out blood from the most distal part of the bowel even without any straining. Very hard stools are often flecked with blood on the surface, apart from which blood can be seen slightly mixed with the faeces. If indeed it is intimately mixed with the stool, the likelihood is that it has come from higher up the bowel. Most commonly, the blood is melancholic or mixed with mucus, then later it is pure red blood. Meanwhile, because it is formed in the empty rectum, it takes the form of a reddish bloodclot, and when indeed there flows from haemorrhoids not blood but slimy material, then it can appropriately be said to be the catarrhal disease, or white discharge from haemorrhoids. (1) (6)

(1) See also Obs. 5.

(6) But what modern authors add is none the less clever. That it is not so much blood which flows, but something like lemon juice or a watery fluid at times. Forestus. *Obs*. 5. Book 23. Schol.

Bayle, on the subject of apoplexy, says he has observed a patient occasionally pass a small piece of material the size of a walnut which was white, glutinous, thick and fibrous, and attached near to the anus. This was evidently a troublesome condition of the rectum, because of which, as it hung down, the patient thought he was having difficulty in passing his stools, and was suffering from sluggishness of the bowels. Bayle thought that this material was coming mainly from haemorrhoids. Bonet. *Anat. Pract*. T. 2. p. 277.

Platerus mentions that this whitish fluid from the haemorrhoidal veins was a substance similar to white of egg. Fernelius also mentions a mucous, whitish, foul discharge. Bonet. Same source.

"In many patients with haemorrhoids there is a distinguishing colour of the whole body, namely lemon-yellow, verging on green". (2) (5)

(2) So says Nicolaus Piso, p. 114.[137]

(5) The colour of a haemorrhoid sufferer's face, according to the evidence of Avicenna, shows this change to be a green hue. Observers of many patients at various times, convinced by this one physical sign, have pronounced them to be suffering from haemorrhoids, with great honour to the profession. Forestus. *Obs*. 5. Book 23.

In addition, where there is bleeding preceded by abdominal colic, it often comes from higher up the bowel. However, it may still come from haemorrhoids if the patient is free of colic. (3)

(3) Not much blood is carried from the mesentery. True blood does not flow from a diseased liver but is diluted rather like the fluid which bathes the flesh of newly slaughtered animals. From torn, bleeding veins of the superior parts, the blood flows dried up and black like pitch. Nicolaus Piso, p. 115.

PROGNOSIS OF HAEMORRHOIDS

The divine Hippocrates affirms that haemorrhoidal bleeding protects mankind from many diseases. *Epidem*. 6. No. 3. Text. 23.[138]

"Those who are wont to bleed from haemorrhoidal vessels are affected neither by pleurisy, nor inflammation of the lungs, nor erosive ulcers (which they call 'phagedaena'), nor furuncles, nor swellings similar to chick peas which they call 'terminthi', nor perhaps even leprosy and other diseases of that sort. Inappropriately, however, many who have been cured have then been attacked by a short illness of this kind, and have been ruinously hit due to the same cause. And this can leave abscesses or fistulae, which are the badge of the stress conditions. And it can be seen from which existing diseases men can be freed and those which they could avert beforehand". He affirms the same theory elsewhere too. V.L. "Dark blood if passed down the bowel is a good thing". *Idem*. 4. Aph. 25.[139]

[137] Nicolaus Piso, *De cognoscendis et curandis praecipue internis humani corporis morbis*, Leiden, O. Visser, 1736, pt 2, book 3, p. 114.

[138] Littré, vol. V. p. 305.

[139] Littré, vol. IV, p. 511.

"Bleeding haemorrhoids prevent incipient black bile and some swelling of the spleen". *Idem.*

Rather it is probable that arthritis itself can be guarded against by passing blood in this way. (4)

(4) As seen in Hist. 6.

IN WHICH ILLNESSES HAEMORRHOIDS HAVE A HEALING EFFECT

Haemorrhoids do not only prevent illness in this way but they can cure many dangerous conditions by bleeding at an appropriate time, as Hippocrates has noted in the passage I have quoted, and the whole medical profession confirms this. One of its members, Boerhaave, who from long and varied experiences must surely be a most learned physician, puts forward the theory that for many diseases this haemorrhoidal bleeding is the one excellent and certain remedy. I have heard him say this in his *Aphorisms*:

"Nephritis is cured in the early stages by a brisk bleed from haemorrhoids". (1)

(1) Boerhaave, Aph. 996, and also Hippocrates: Haemorrhoids following depression and nephritis are most valuable. 6 Aph.[140]

"Bleeding from haemorrhoidal swellings often supervenes and brings a cure" (that is, on speaking about depression). (2)

(2) Boerhaave, Aph. 1110.[141]

"A slight stroke can be relieved by a copious, long-lasting bleed from haemorrhoids". (3)

(3) Id. Aph. 996.[142]

"When attempts by every known cure have failed in mania, haemorrhoidal varices occurring later can be of value". (4)

(4) Id. Aph. 1124.[143] Hippocrates confirms that if haemorrhoids or rectal varices develop in insane patients, then the insanity is relieved. 6. Aph. 21. Id. speaking of the onset of menstruation.[144]

"He states in passing that he has seen the most unbelievable example of this (5), and we should imitate him before including these unfortunates for life among the incurables".

(5) See Obs. 12.6.

"He teaches that varicose veins and bleeding haemorrhoids are good for delirious and frantic patients (6) and, as a cure for frenzy, he recommends provoking a flow of blood by bathing the anus, by rubbing the haemorrhoids with fig leaves and by suction by leeches". (7)

[140] Boerhaave, *Aphorismi*, p. 225; Littré, vol. VI, p. 569.
[141] Ibid., p. 261.
[142] Ibid., p. 225.
[143] Ibid., p. 263.
[144] Littré, vol. IV, p. 569.

(6) Boerhaave, Aph. 702 and 779.[145] Also Hippocrates.
(7) Id. Aph. 781.[146]

Fortunately innumerable other ailments can be cured by this health-giving evacuation of blood, such as epileptic dizziness, distention with wind, diseases of the hypochondria, jaundice, cirrhosis of the liver and spleen, inflammation of the uterus and genitals, scurvy and quartan fevers. The authors give examples throughout their writings and, because of their particular value, these veins are termed "golden".

On rare occasions this loss of blood is harmful, but in most cases it is absolutely useful and necessary, so that Hippocrates notes "if anyone wants to arrest long-lasting haemorrhoids, unless he allows one vessel to bleed, he runs the risk of oedema or disease". Galen also reminds us "not a few depressed patients are made insane by the arrest of haemorrhoidal bleeding, others develop pleurisy, and yet others oedema". Nay rather, when haemorrhoidal bleeding ceases inopportunely, the materia peccans is often transferred to the liver, spleen, lungs or brain and causes obstructions and hard inflammation of these parts to some extent. And so this type of patient becomes the victim of all those ailments which could be cured by haemorrhoidal bleeding at the right moment, before they show themselves. Besides, these cases are often afflicted by leg ulcers, carcinoma, arthritis, nose-bleeding and haemoptysis, and truly almost all the leading physicians speak out on the subject and experience throughout the ages gives a massive confirmation of their views. The great Stahl, Professor of Medicine at Halle and founder of a large school of medical men, is in no way to be considered wrong when he states (according to my information) that fever is a part of natural motive force which tries to deposit the evil humours into the haemorrhoidal vessels and by the same principle, it derives the special origin of all ills from the noxious material of which haemorrhoids appear to be the natural means of disposal.

HAEMORRHOIDAL BLEEDING IS SOMETIMES HARMFUL

When this outflow is untimely and not critical, but due to weakness of the haemorrhoidal vessels or from too much irritation; or when the blood flow is excessive, and valuable blood is lost after a bad humour has been expelled, then it is a cause of various diseases. Then, the patients become pale and utterly weak and first show the weakness in the legs and sometimes bleeding haemorrhoids can deprive them of life; this is of course when serious haemorrhage or oedema develop. Cirrhosia, carcinoma or gangrene arise from severe inflammation, indeed most often an abscess is produced which on account of its natural situation is easily and very quickly turned into an anal fistula, which is very difficult to cure. So that these warnings may become clearer and well-known, it will be necessary briefly to set forth the origin, cause, nature and uses of the special blood vessels near the anus, the explanation of which I often consider most strikingly helps nature.

[145] Boerhaave, *Aphorismi*, pp. 140, 161.
[146] Ibid., p. 161.

ON THE CONSTRUCTION AND PURPOSE OF HAEMORRHOIDAL VESSELS

Shortly after the portal veins divide into two main branches, one important internal haemorrhoidal vein emerges from the so-called splenic vein, and its branches are widely dispersed in a very tortuous manner throughout the mesentery, first of all to the large colon and eventually ending in great abundance in the rectum. It is likely there are less conspicuous branches which up to now have not been examined closely by the anatomists in an authoritative way, also reaching the anus. At times, this vein arises from the right branch of the portal vein or from the angle between the bifurcation. (1)

(1) These variations in structure are best described by Eustachius in his Tab. 27 [*sic*] & Figs. 2 & 4; however they are also sketched by Verhein along with the portal system. Tab. 39. Fig 2.g.[147]

The inferior mesenteric artery moreover approaches this vein, taking bile with it to the bifurcation of the haemorrhoidal vein. (2)

(2) See Eustachius. Ibid.

This branch also goes off to supply the rectum and approaches the internal haemorrhoidal vessel. The hypogastric vein and artery give off some branches to the rectum, others to the bladder, the genital organs, the nearby muscles of the buttocks and finally, some called the external haemorrhoidal vessels supply the anus. (3)

(3) Eustachius Tab. [*sic*] 13 and Verhein Tab. 39. Fig 1.e.[148]

Some authors state that the branches from the sacral vein and artery also supply the anus. (5)

(5) See Nicolaus Piso.

It must also be said that the course of the internal haemorrhoidal vessels is very tortuous, and by this means the vessels reach out to the farthest limits of the portal system. As a result, the haemorrhoidal veins are much larger than any other branches of the portal vessels (4) and because of the erect posture of the human body, the blood coursing through them attains a much greater height than through the other mesenteric vessels.

(4) Eustachius drew these veins most beautifully.

ON HAEMORRHOIDS

It is indeed noteworthy that the internal haemorrhoidal veins and all the mesenteric veins are supplied with small valves, as Ruysch first demonstrated by means of his wonderful injection technique. Thus, the blood is easily pumped through these veins both upwards and downwards, so that greater pressure is applied to one part than to another. Besides, these veins most often communicate with each other by anastomoses so that fluid can flow to and fro from one part through all the rest. If therefore any cause of some strength impedes the free flow of the blood to the liver, then because of the abundant orifices of the mesenteric veins, the impeded blood is distributed through the entire mesenteric system quickly and equally, which is absolutely necessary. Just as the blood is

[147] Bartholomaeus Eustachius, *Opuscula anatomica*, Venice, V. Luchinus, 1564, it should read Tab. 2, p. 7; Philip Verheyen, *Corporis humani anatomia libri*, Brussels, Serstevens, 1726, p. 382.

[148] Ibid., but, in the first reference, Brownrigg is referring to page, not tabula, 13 of *Opuscula anatomica*.

driven from the limbs, first through the returning veins by two forces, that is by the muscles which serve animal motion and then by the contractile force of the heart and arteries, so this occurs in the mesenteric veins also. By alternating contraction of the diaphragm and abdominal muscles, these vessels are compressed and blood is driven towards the liver. But on contemplating the construction and situation of the haemorrhoidal veins it will become clear that the arrival of the blood into them is somewhat assisted by the action of the respiratory muscles; indeed, because of this it is more impeded by complete compression of these veins so that the propulsion of the blood attempting to contrive its usual action succeeds brilliantly. The haemorrhoidal vessels therefore lack this muscular strength by which, remarkably, the flow of blood is pumped to other parts of the body. Another force which propels the flow of blood throughout the mesenteric veins is the circular motion of arterial blood which is pumped, according to this principle, into the veins. But the velocity of the arterial fluid is greatly slowed down when the internal haemorrhoidal veins often open into the farthermost parts of the system, to the great advantage of nature, and by this easy rapid means, the whole body can be rid of foul, dark bile and melancholic humours. On the same principle the innumerable diseases of the abdominal organs can be abolished or at least guarded against, and countless defects of the brain, lungs and skin can be cured solely by the transfer of the peccant material from the affected parts to the haemorrhoidal area. It is possible for untold numbers of illnesses to be drawn out of the system when the noxious humours deposited there are channelled to the more noble parts of the body. Besides, it is clear that the blood flow in the external haemorrhoidal veins is more useful in many diseases than in the internal ones. It is possible that from the anastomoses of the internal vessels with the external ones or from the course of the internal vessels to those on the exterior, the internal haemorrhoidal vessels may be emptied through the opening of the external. Nay, indeed, the external haemorrhoidal vessels, like the uterine, take their origin in the first place from the hypogastric vessels, whence the same healing effects ought to follow of necessity from the opening of the external haemorrhoidal vessels as much as from that of the uterine vessels. This explains how the haemorrhoidal veins because of their situation and special anatomical construction are most eminently suitable for the separating out and the disposal of the evil humours. Indeed, it is clear as much from theoretical reasoning as from practical experience, that these veins are often opened greatly to the benefit and profit of mankind. By this natural disposal of evil substances, amazing results can be achieved by nature which are very worthy of imitation by the medical profession. It is indeed rare for haemorrhoidal bleeding to be harmful, nor should it be thought easily arrested without first pondering very carefully the constitution of the patient, the present illness, or those which might well follow.[149]

[Three small inserted pages.]

1

On excessive haemorrhoidal bleeding—see Harris—on acute illnesses in infants. Book 2. Obs. 10.[150]

[149] This lengthy dissertation on haemorrhoids reflects Brownrigg's own thoughts on the condition. He shows himself to be acquainted with both the ancient theories and also the current ideas among most members of his profession in the eighteenth century. It is possible he may have intended to publish this discourse.

[150] Walter Harris, *De morbis acutis infantum*, Amsterdam, J. F. Bernard, 1715, p. 187.

[The following is part of a page torn from a book-seller's catalogue.]
308 Sydenham de podagra . . .
309 Waldschmidi instit. med. 1645
310 Silvii praxis medica 1674 quatuor libri
311 Willis Cerebri Anatomia 1664
312 Pineus de Virginitate 1650
313 Hartmanni prax. Chimiatri 1647
314 Harvaei de motu Cordis 1661
315 . . . . . . 1662 duo libri.

2

On haemorrhoids—In the section on the treatment. See Marcellus Donatus. de Mirab. page 581. Also Boerhaave. Historia—Rare cases not previously described.[151]

3

On haemorrhoids: writings.
Sanctorius in his Opuscul Med.
Stahl. See tract on haemorrhoids: ditto, his own true Medicine.
Dr. Mich. Alberti. On haemorrhoids.
Hales 1772 Quarto. lfl. 10 kr.[152]

[Small sheets of paper pasted in.]

The following are my own observations:

Mrs. Copeland, a widow, after a serious episode of depression at about the time of her 43rd year, completely ceased to menstruate for two whole years and this led to a poor appetite, morning sickness, loss of weight and hysterical affections. The vomiting might perhaps have taken the place of her menstrual periods, as it does in pregnant women. About the beginning of February 1740 her external haemorrhoids began to swell up, causing her to suffer severe pain, then they began to bleed and for a short time her hysterical affections and back pain ceased, and then afterwards the periods recommenced.

Mrs. Wylde, a woman aged 42, blessed with a robust constitution, gave birth to a daughter during the first few years after her marriage. The lochia did not flow properly. After that she menstruated twice and then during the first year after conceiving again, indeed in the third week after a serious illness, she brought up a considerable quantity of mucous fluid. For the rest of her time, though quite fit in herself, she was cruelly troubled by a skin rash on her arm, which on examination had the appearance of herpes.

Captain Lutwidge, a 60-year-old man. For many years he had suffered from intermittent diarrhoea and because of this he had had relief from several ailments. Also in this winter of

[151] Marcellus Donatus, *De historia medica mirabili*, Frankfurt, E. Kempffer for J. J. Porsius, 1613, bk 5, p. 581. Hermann Boerhaave, *Atrocis nec descripti prius, morbi historia altera*, Leiden, S. Luchtmans, T. Haak, 1728.

[152] Giovanni Santorini, *Opuscula medica de structu & motu fibrae*, Rotterdam, 1719. Georg Ernst Stahl, *De motu haemorrhoidali, et fluxu haemorrhoidum*, Paris, 1730; *Theoria medica vera*, Halle, 1708, 2nd ed. 1721. Chapters X–XIII, pp. 309–27, in Michael Alberti's *Introductio in medicinam*, Halle, Orphanotropheum, 1721, deals with haemorrhoids. The reference to Hales has not been identified.

1740 he had copious bleeding from internal haemorrhoids, but I postively refused to stem the flow since I knew that he would be cured of his hypochondria and other hysterical affections.

Master George Spedding, aged about 20, was a sufferer from rickets which made him thin, with a crooked body and a narrow chest. Moreover he often suffered from rectal prolapse. In the autumn of 1739 he had been suffering for 7 or 8 weeks from severe colic. Then, when the colic stopped, he passed a quantity of watery, serous blood after moving his bowels, and even when he had not done so, three, four or five times a day. This caused him frequent pains in his back, weakness, loss of weight and thirst. Therefore when I realised that the bleeding was the cause of his weakness I ordered that it should be curbed with medicines which would staunch the flow and make him stronger, and I prescribed the following:

Bolus with rhubarb, then an electuary with bloodstone, Peruvian bark, Fracastor's confection, sugar and squills. Make up with 3 spoonfuls of red sandalwood and tormentil. With this treatment he became well again.

Captain How, a soldier, robust and of strong constitution, the son of a father restricted by arthritis, and much addicted to the joys of Bacchus and Venus. This was a man in his forties and for many years past he had been much tormented by hereditary joint pains and he had had two long episodes of this illness in 1738. In the autumn of that year his internal haemorrhoids bled freely with pure, florid but useful blood and he scarcely noticed the first attack of pain. There is a remarkable case of his brother Peter How—a similar case indeed like the remarkable case of Mrs. Wylde.

Mr. Bowman, a man in his fifties, had been suffering every year from slight arthritis after severe depression and serious attacks of rage. He changed his way of life, nor could he return to it while his joint pains were uncontrolled. He had violent sickness with fever, poor appetite and thirst. I prescribed a dose of Thae Sacra. His external haemorrhoids swelled up, his symptoms vanished, and that winter he had no trouble from his arthritis. He was ordered to take a bitter electuary as a tonic with the same type of wine.

[Small page inserted.][153]

Bow.

This farm labourer aged 20, usually in the best of health, caught a cold about Christmas time. About the beginning of February he developed chest pains with sweating in the mornings and these symptoms persisted for six to eight weeks, accompanied by abdominal colic. Then a most terrible headache seized him which was greatly aggravated by exercise, stooping and coughing, with vertigo at the end of each attack. Pains remained fixed in one place, like the Clavus hystericus. That week he noticed serious clouding of vision. Objects 200-feet away appeared double at all times but at shorter distances they were single. If he

[153] Brownrigg appears to have inserted this small page here for no reason; likewise the following two prescriptions for patients already described earlier in the Casebook.

looked with only one eye, they were still single. Small pulse, weak and rapid; cough with frothy white sputum; breathing quite freely; bowels normal; appetite fair; no severe thirst; tongue coated.

Objects appeared double due to muscular contraction. Vision clouded by damage to the nerves. Headache is due to cerebral infarction and nervous ataxia. The humours are to be diverted from the brain by cautery, shaving the head, footbaths and gentle purgatives. Rehabilitate the strength with an easily digestible diet. Gentle exercise. Electuary of ground myrrh, saffron, etc., to be taken in milk twice daily, at breakfast and supper.

Mr. Thompson. [Case No. 45. Repeat of the prescription. Perhaps the original rough note.]

Mr. Dan. [Case No. 48. Also a rough note of the prescriptions.]

1738

70 Mr. Allen, suffering from ascites, due to jaundice.

This man was about 50 years old, of spare constitution, active, keen witted and of stiff fibre. He had worked for 26 years as an excise officer. Has led a temperate life, but for three years he has been drinking a lot of wine, mostly punch. He had enjoyed excellent health practically all his life, except when he had bad jaundice thirty years ago and also an attack of intermittent fever nine years ago. Both these episodes rapidly cleared up with treatment.

June. In the month of June last, after a strenuous drinking bout which lasted all night, he felt ill and developed a slight fever, with pain in his side and a very dry tongue. These symptoms disappeared within a day or two, then his skin became jaundiced, his stools became pale in colour, and his forces were considerably weakened. He took various remedies for the jaundice and the condition somewhat improved, then after another drinking session at the end of August, he once more developed a fever, with sharp pain in his side aggravated by breathing. His tongue became very dry and coated with deep fissures on the surface and his abdomen was greatly distended with wind. I was called at this stage and bled him at once. The blood was thin and runny with inflammatory crusts on it. After using nitrous mixture with syrup of tamarind and rob. of elderflower and rhubarb purges with saline cathartic apozems, the fever went away, but he remained weak and, to eliminate the icteric cacochymy, I prescribed gummous pills, but he refused to take them in spite of the fact that his abdomen swelled perceptibly as a result.

November 12th. I was called in again and noted the following symptoms: pulse regular but rapid, very small and weak; respiration satisfactory, but moving about and his swollen abdomen made breathing difficult; tongue moist ; appetite good; occasional thirst during the night; bowels moving normally; stools now the normal colour.

Nov. 12th, 1738.
The illness is ? dropsy and jaundice from destruction of the liver. Indications for cure—these must include relief of obstructions, elimination of stagnant fluids and the resumption of bodily strength. An easily digestible diet must be given and frequent drying frictions must be commenced. Heat should be passed to the body from a fire and applications.

Best saffron 1 scruple; Ammoniac gum 2½ scruples; Venetian soap ½ oz; Juniper oil 15 drops; Sassafras oil 15 drops. Strassburg turpentine, enough to make up 12 pills, each of 1 scruple. Take 1 every hour of the day, followed by 2 spoonfuls of:
Centaury leaves 1 peck; Hypericum leaves 1 peck; Root of turmeric ½ oz; Tincture of madder ½ oz; Root of sea holly ½ oz; Juniper berries 3 oz; Orange flavouring 1 scruple; Wormwood ½ scruple. Boil gently in a closed vessel for 1 hour with spring water to make 2 pts. Strain, divide, squeeze and then allow to settle, then add:
Juniper spirit 2 oz; Weak wormwood 2 oz.

He was passing large amounts of urine which was dark red with a light, whitish flocculent sediment and of a most beautiful colour. Moderate swelling on the side of the shins. Skin yellowish, tinged with green; the whites of his eyes also somewhat yellowish-green; swelling of thighs most noticeable towards evening but disappearing in the mornings; abdomen distended and hard, indeed as tight as a drum; swelling of irregular size.

I later prescribed the following:

Fresh bardan root 3 oz; Parsley root 3 oz; Root of sea holly 3 scruples; Root of flowering iris 3 scruples; Root of elecampane 3 scruples; Root of angelica 3 scruples; All the herbs and dandelion ½ pt; Juniper berries 3 oz. Boil gently for ¼ hr in a closed flask with spring water. Make up 3 pts. Strain and strongly squeeze, then add: Radish water 4 oz; Pure nitre ½ oz; Rob. of elderflower 2 oz. Take 4 spoonfuls every 2 hours.
Take 10 drops of nitre spirit in a single dose.

[Additional marginal note.]

Fed up with this treatment, he betook himself to another doctor. The heavy fees attached by a huge examination and prescriptions pained him, so he took several pastilles urged on him by old wives, but without effect, for his abdomen was daily becoming still more distended until death put an end to his misery.

September 10th, 1737

71 Thomas Stoker, died of dropsy. This sailor was a robust and temperate man in his forties, who had been suffering for about two months from a fever with a cough which had started after he had caught a cold. His fever had now gone, but his breathing was quite laboured and wheezy and much more difficult when he lay down in bed than when he was sitting up. Cough small and dry; pulse poor in volume and weak; abdomen swollen all over and more or less distended. His thighs were greatly swollen and pitted on digital pressure; his legs swelled towards night-time. He had no appetite. Urine scanty and thickened with a sediment like brickdust. Thirsty.

Venetian turpentine 6 scruples; Whisk up 2 egg yolks and add: Ammoniac gum 2 scruples; Myrrh gum 2 scruples; Gum mastic 2 scruples; Honey 2 oz. Make an electuary the size of a nutmeg and take 4 times per day.
Make a mixture of the following and take 3 spoonfuls:
Strong cinnamon water 6 oz; Oxymel of squills 4 oz; Tincture of saffron 2 scruples; Spirit of lavender 2 scruples.

One week later. Respiration easier but cough very troublesome with some sputum. Increased abdominal swelling. I prescribed pills with small beer.

> Gum ammoniac 1 scruple; Myrrh 1 scruple; Gum mastic; Benzoin flower ½ scruple; Wormwood ½ scruple; Venetian soap 2 scruples; Extract of liquorice 2 scruples; Aniseed oil 20 drops; Juniper oil 20 drops; Peruvian bark. Make up pills of 5 gr. Take 4 four times a day. Follow with a drink of small beer—8 spoonfuls.

Two weeks later. Pulse slight and irregular in every way; breathing a little easier; sweating and abdominal swelling slightly less. Because of the urgent requests of those at his bedside, I prescribed a cathartic of black mechoacan root and syrup of thorns which was repeated every three hours as his strength was utterly gone, but his swelling and other symptoms improved very little. In addition then I prescribed an electuary, a remedy which did not suit the patient at all.

> Herbs 2 pecks; Hyssop 2 pecks; Pennyroyal 2 pecks; Ivy 2 pecks; Angelica root 2 oz; Elecampane root 2 oz; Iris root 2oz; Juniper berries ½ pt. Pour into strong beer to make up 6 pints.

At the request of his friends I also ordered wine with gin, but all these medicaments were of no avail and he died about the end of October.

> Root of fresh chives 2 oz; Elecampane root 2 oz; Red radish root 2 oz; Cardamon sugar 4 oz. Pound together in a mortar and add: Birthwort root 2 scruples; Flowering iris root 2 scruples; Zedoar root 2 scruples; Tartar salt 1½ scruples; Juniper oil 30 drops. Take a piece the size of a nutmeg every 2 hours.

Early May, 1738

72 Mrs. Beck of Cockermouth, died of dropsy due to jaundice. A woman in her fifties who had lived in Spain for twenty years. She had been single all her life, living in luxury on rich foods and strong wines from Alicante. She was of stout constitution, verging on obesity. Last winter she developed, as it seemed to me, epidemic inflammatory fever and with a view to curing this she had unwisely taken Peruvian bark. She then gradually became dropsical and in order to rid herself of the fluid she had taken repeated doses of cathartics, but with unfortunate results as a review of her symptoms will show. Pulse rapid and weak; breathing laboured so that she was unable to lie flat. She could not get out of bed because of great prostration. She was bringing up thick sputum almost continually and had frequent attacks of nausea and vomiting and she could swallow nothing except bread saps or fruit juices with wine. Insatiable thirst; bowels normal; urine scanty and thick; skin yellow in colour; marked abdominal swelling, but it was not uniform and was greatest in the hypochondria; no swelling of legs; sleepless.

Query—Is this condition dropsy with ascites associated with hydratid swellings? Are its remote causes her age and the fact that she has spent the last six years of her life in a cooler climate than before? Is it preposterous to treat inflammatory conditions of the blood with Peruvian bark? Is the proximate cause of illness obstruction of the liver? Mr. Clementson relates the history of a young girl who suffered from ascites and was cured of the condition when treated by blisters applied to the abdomen, when a large quantity of fluid was drained off. Do these epispastics help the breathing, or do they increase the thirst and fever too much and bring on gangrene? So therefore it is not at all safe to try such remedies which are untried and uncertain in effect. Should cathartics be used? In this case they were tried and were useless, leading to weakness of the patient and so I was unwilling to continue using them any longer. Certainly cathartics do not help, indeed they are very harmful by increasing fever and thirst with their sharpness, weakening the patient's vigour and natural strength, destroying the obstructed blood vessels and causing the stagnant humours to become putrid. The greatest quantity of fluid can be observed in bladder obstruction when it becomes extremely difficult to pass the stream of urine. If, however, the illness does not yield to such evacuants, then emetics might be more suitable as these would seem to affect more closely the seat of the disease.

With the aim of strengthening the body, relieving the thirst, opening the fluid channels and either absorbing the excess fluids into the body or dissipating them by means of the urine or perspiration, I prescribed various remedies, but without success, for the patient remained very ill for six or seven weeks and then died. After her death, Mr. Clementson, by performing a paracentesis, drained about six pints of fluid like water in which meat has been washed. He estimated that the abdomen still contained another 6 pints of fluid, but he had not been able to drain it through the incision he had made. The treatments I used are here described:

Mrs. Beck—remedies for dropsy
Using a drying diet with small, strong drinks thus:
Rhenish or Alicante wine with some drops of spirit of sweet nitre. Her abdomen must be strongly rubbed every day, as much as her skin can allow.
Herb of whole crushed dandelion 1 pt; Juniper berries ½ pt; Root of cut flowering iris 3 scruples; Root of elecampane 3 scruples; Vitriolated tartar 1 scruple; Rhenish wine generously aged 2 pts; Juniper spirit 1 oz.
Dissolve together in a bain-marie with costmary for 3 hrs. Strain and strongly squeeze. Take 2 spoonfuls every 2 hrs.
To relieve the thirst, chew mastic.
To move and corroborate the stomach, make a poultice of Andromachus treacle with a little turpentine and wormwood oil.
Herbs: Fresh broadleaved wormwood 1 peck; Fumitory 1 peck; Brooklime 1 peck.
Cut off, slice, pound and express the juices into a single draught. Add 1½ oz white sugar and after boiling gently, filter through a conical bag of cotton and store in a cool place until required.
4 oz of the prescribed juice: Juniper spirit 3 scruples; Tincture of black hellebore from the *London Pharmacopoeia* 1½ scruples; Tincture of myrrh 1 scruple; Elixir of myrrhic vitriol 30 drops; Sal martis 1 scruple; Rob. of juniper 3 scruples.
Take 1 oz at 6, 7, 8, 10 and 11 in the morning every day.[154]

[Inserted later into the margin of Mrs. Beck's case is the following:]

73 *1738*

Mrs. Grave of Keswick, a woman of 50 with eight children. Last winter her periods ceased altogether. About the beginning of June, after catching a cold, she felt severe pain and swelling and distention of the hypochondrium. She tried various remedies but the illness increased day by day and fluid collected within her abdomen.

[154] Mrs. Beck—yet another alcoholic who developed jaundice and ascites, confirmed at the post mortem.

30th September. I saw her and noted the following symptoms: pulse weak, rapid and irregular; respiration very laboured so that she was obliged to sit up in a chair all day and all night; very troublesome cough with bloodstained or ichorous sputum; could not bear the sight of food; tremendous thirst; urine scanty and reddish-brown in colour with heavy sediment. Severe continuous pain in the hypochondria going through to the back, worse on the left side than the right; swelling in the abdomen large and hard; legs and thighs incredibly thickened by fluid in the skin.

I predicted that all remedies would be useless, and she indeed died ten or twelve days later.

[The following has only the latter part of the case copied into the Casebook, perhaps an oversight on Brownrigg's part?]

February 15th, 1737/8

74 Mrs. Widdow Kelsick.

. . . after pressing with a finger, indentations were left behind. The disease was seen to be a watery growth on the ligament of her big toe, and some of the membranes which were affected round it gave her great pain from their swelling. The growth on her toe does not retain a mark when pressed, nor is it extended to the whole leg. The matter does not confine itself within cell-like membranes as in an anasarca. The congested matter is full of phlegm, sluggish and thick. The following indications may show how to cure this: to disperse the congested material and to prevent any fresh accumulation; to take care of the lungs and not to weaken the bile and blood-forming organs.

See the remedy shown described on the previous page.

After this she was regularly seized with all the true spasms of arthritis.

Fresh root of wild radish 4 scruples; Elecampane root 4 scruples; Flowering iris root 4 scruples; Angelica root 4 scruples; Hyssop root 4 scruples; Zedoar root 2 scruples; Orange peel 3 scruples; Juniper berries 3 oz; Sweet fennel seed 3 scruples; Mustard seed 3 scruples; Cochineal 2 scruples; Old Rhenish wine 4 pts; Tincture of salt of tartar 1 oz. Pound together to produce a tincture.

Leaves of common wormwood 2 pecks; St. John's wort 6 pecks; Root of elecampane 6 scruples; Angelica root 6 scruples; Sassafras wood shavings 2 oz; seed of wild carrot 2 oz; Juniper berries 8 oz.

Chop up, pound and mix. Place in a bag and mix with fresh small beer. Make up 6 pts, then she is to drink it regularly as her ordinary drink.

February 20th, 1737/8

75 Mr. Peile of Cockermouth, suffering from anasarca and perhaps a chest dropsy. A man of 42 who lost a leg 6 years ago, of sanguine constitution but an active and indefatigable drinker and he indulged in spirituous liquors to excess. For six months he had suffered from a great weakness of the stomach, he rejected food to the extent that his life was only supported by his strong drinks. These symptoms, sleeplessness, and all the excesses were increased at the time of the Election.[155] Symptoms: pulse slight, fast and irregular; no dry

[155] A political election in Cockermouth, where Sir James Lowther was a dominant figure.

heat of fever; breathing difficult and quite small, and in an asthmatic manner; frequent heart palpitations; a troublesome cough without phlegm; very great weakness. His appetite was almost wholly destroyed and he vomited anything at meals, but could retain with immense feelings of illness vinous liquors and other strong drinks. His urine was a little reddish in colour with a great deal of sediment. He had fluid in the legs and he did not sleep. His stools were those of a healthy man, and his colour was good.

Firstly, to restore the vitality of the chyle-producing organs, to improve the necessary digestive processes, to prevent the irregularity of the nerves, to improve the evacuations, to remove the obstructions, I prescribed various remedies. An electuary of bitter-tasting corroborants. A bitter aromatic wine and pills of gum with soap. All these were of no use as his stomach rejected all the remedies attempted and he perished last month.

DISSERTATION

The illness of dropsy as a result of drinking is frequently very difficult to cure, for the sufferers are weak and often no medical treatment can clear the obstruction once the chyle-producing organs are totally destroyed. In private lectures, the distinguished Siegfried Albinus cut into the body of a dropsical woman who had suffered and died from abuse of spirituous liquors. He found two heavy stones about 3 scruples and ½ oz in her bile duct, one of these was conical and the other fitted into the hollow of its base. The passage disappeared above and below this into a ligament and the liver was hardened into a friable mass. Moreover, the stomach was curled and dried in such a strange manner that it would scarcely have held anything the size of a walnut. In many bodies, after long illness, I have noted that the adipose pannicle is filled with a yellow ichorous humour instead of fat.

[This is a letter to his former tutor at Leiden, Gerhard van Swieten, before the latter's departure to Vienna].

Mr. Richard Kelsick, Jnr.

To the most excellent and learned J. Van Sueten, M.D. W. Brownrigg, Sender.

76 Mr. R. K., a sailor of 21, of slight build and with a thin body. His father suffered from general rheumatic pains and irregular spells of arthritis, and his mother had inherited an arthritic condition from his grandfather. From boyhood he had frequently been troubled by vague rheumatic pains. Two years ago he went in a ship to the British colony of Virginia and stayed there until the beginning of September last year. In August he began to suffer from tertian fever, which is a common illness in these regions, often serious and with many dying from it. After three or four weeks the tertian fever assumed a regularity, and to remove this, after proper consultation, he swallowed excessive amounts of Peruvian bark at times. As long as he used this, the fever was kept away, but it recurred after 10 or 12 days until the illness died away at the end of last May.

However, after the fever had been checked 2 or 3 times by Peruvian bark in November of last year, his feet began to swell and he was severely tormented by this misery. I went to see him very recently and noted that the swelling occupied the ankles and extended along the bones to the foot and toes. The swelling appeared white and resistant to finger pressure. Although the swelling was very considerable it was not accompained by pain or heat and the greatest amount was in the back of the feet. A little pain was felt below his outer ankle bones by finger pressure, but when he stood up he was scarcely able to walk on account of the great tenderness and weakness of the soles of his feet, unless he was supported by small sticks. Since then, the swelling and softness has spread to the big toes and through the long bones of the main metatarsals, then to other parts. His feet have contracted and curved in on the outer parts so that he stands on his little toes. Moreover his feet are constantly wet with moisture and the veins under the skin are very swollen. Such is the nature of the swelling. Last summer once, he passed copious fresh blood from internal haemorrhoids and other causes. I do not know what kind of effect caused it, or if this evacuation would remedy this swelling, so that is why I consult you. His skin colour turns yellowish which may in part be a result of the inclement weather. He has recovered well in other respects. At present I have prescribed liniment A and wine B with wholesome food and exercise. I will make certain that no other ingredients or remedies will be given to relieve the swelling until you have sent your opinion on its nature. Therefore I eagerly await your advice with which, as in all your cases, I will be most grateful and will find most useful for my patient.

Farewell.

Written Whitehaven
3/12 1738. By the old Reckoning.[156]

I wish to be commended to the very distinguished Dr. Gronovius, M.D. A few fossils and especially the iron minerals dug up in Cumberland are sent with this note.

A. Spirit of salt 1½ oz; Vinegar 5 oz; Venetian soap 6 scruples; Tincture of castor ½ oz; Camphor ½ scruple. Mix together. Rub the feet once morning and night for half an hour using a warm, dry woollen cloth and then anoint the swelling with the liniment described above, adding pork dripping.

B. Root of Angelica ½ oz; Root of hyssop ½ oz; Virginian snake root ½ oz; Sassafras bark 2½ scruples; Winter's bark 1 scruple; Cochineal 1 scruple; Old Rhenish wine 2 pts; Salt of wormwood 3 scruples. Boil in a closed vessel to make up the wine. Take 2 spoonfuls 4 times a day on an empty stomach.

[The following is not the original letter, but is copied in Brownrigg's hand into the Casebook.]

To the very learned and wise Dr. W. Brownrigg from the hand of J. Van Swieten.

I have carefully thought about the case you have described and here set down my opinion. Having suppressed the fever so many times and not having cured it, in order to effect a cure, an attempt must be made to move the sluggish material of the illness into parts less resistant and less troubled by this way of life, possibly also if they are already weakened by heredity. Note that clearing out the blood through the bowels without pain or straining seems to be as a result of the mesentery vessels which free themselves from the

[156] While the Continent had changed over to the Gregorian calendar, Britain still retained the old Julian method at this date, and Brownrigg is drawing Van Swieten's attention to this.

pressing blood, while perhaps the transmission of abdominal blood through the liver has been less effective. To cure the affliction I should recommend the following:

Diet of easily digestible foods, especially a substantial amount of vegetables. Weakening drinks of warm water should be avoided, but a moderate amount of vintage wine or neat beer might help.

Every morning and evening for a quarter of an hour, the feet must be held in vapour rising from incense, then gently rubbed with flannels penetrated by the same vapour.

Take 3 pills B. every 3 hours daily after a drink. 4 oz of the decoction C. Although the winter weather is unfavourable, I dare to hope for a favourable outcome to this matter.

Farewell, I am your

J. Van Swieten.

Written Leyden, 23 December, 1738.

A. Amber 1 oz; Strax 1 scruple; Calamint 1 scruple; Olibanum 1 scruple; Gum mastic 1 scruple; Benzoin 1 scruple. Make powders of 1 or 2 scruples. Sprinkle them on glowing coals.

B. Root of best rhubarb 1½ scruples; Root of saffron ½ scruple; Opopanax gum 1 scruple; Giant fennel gum 1 scruple; Venetian soap; Common turpentine. Make up pills of 4 gr.

C. Root of sweet radish. Boil in ordinary water for half an hour and add: Bark 1 oz; Sandalwood 1 oz; Sassafras 2 oz; Salt polychrest 2 scruples.
After boiling together in a closed flask for half an hour, strain and administer 3 pts of the liquid.

[The remainder is Brownrigg's observation after following Van Swieten's cure.]

The above described were used for three months and relieved this illness and he was able to walk without the use of a stick, however, the tenderness and weakness remained and also the swelling already noted in the feet and ankle bones. About 20th March he was seized by ophthalmia in the whole eye. The white was entirely red, the eye was hot and he was affected by continual headaches and a stabbing, lancing pain which grew more severe at night. The illness appeared again very severely and to it were added the torments of scrofula and oedematous growths noted by Maître Jean.[157]

His tongue was white and the pulse strong and irregular, causing him great trouble. Leeches were applied to the temples three or four times and blood taken from his arm the same number of times. He took purgative drinks on alternate days and in the intervening time used cold, salty laxative and antiphlogistic remedies and a light diet. Poultices and various eye salves were applied to the affected eye, but notwithstanding these remedies his illness continued on to the end of May. By that time there were suppurations from the cheekbones, by which surprisingly he was alleviated in a week or two from his illness. Moreover, his feet which had remained weak during the course of treatment began to grow stronger as the humour began to subside. When the eye condition . . .

[157] Perhaps a reference to a learned work, but the doctor has not been traced.

[The rest of this case history is obscured by the following note in English pasted over it:]

If you should chance to be at any time affected as formerly. If the Inflammation in your Eye it will be proper to have ten or twelve ounces of blood drawn from your Arm or from the Jugular Vein once, twice, oftner or seldomer according to the Violence of the Inflammation & fever which attends it and according as your Strength will permit. Leeches applyed to your Temples may also be of some Service. It will likewise be necessary to take some Cooling Purges every second or third day as you have conveniency, repeating them untill the disorder begins to abate. For this Purpose the purging Ingredients are directed. A Paper of which Ingredients two spoonfuls of the purging mixture. On the intermediate days when you do not make use of the Purges Take the Quantity of a Nutmeg of the Cooling and Opening Electuary drinking a draught of the Barley Water. Collyrium.
Directions given to Mr. Kelsick going to Sea.

December 1738

77 Mrs. Hudelstone[158] dying of Puerperal Fever. A woman, properly virtuous and keeping to the mean in the fabric and temperament of her body. She gave birth a year ago, for the first time, and her lochia were totally suppressed from that time. Thereafter she suffered from a white flux until the beginning of this pregnancy and from the cessation of her periods and from other serious symptoms and has been totally prostrate until her death, with cruel colic pains, and her urine was rank and mixed with foul material and passed with severe pain.

Day 1. Date of the birth 29 November.

In the evening, after coming to the correct term of her pregnancy, she gave birth to a strong and lively girl. The midwife was in fact timid and not very experienced and could not remove all the afterbirth carefully, as the placenta had adhered to the left side of the uterus too strongly. A surgeon was called. On account of the contraction of the uterus he could not introduce his hand; however, by working his fingers into the uterus, he separated the placenta and removed the afterbirth. As he reported, the placenta seemed to be a little torn and also very tender, and he freely confessed, on account of the contraction, some of the placenta had perhaps remained in the uterus.

Day 2. She was cheerful after the birth, but next day she felt a very violent pain in the area of the adhesion of the placenta.

Day 3. She was afflicted by the same pains, which were a little reduced by the application of anodynes. Meanwhile the lochia responded.

Day 4. About noon I was called in and noted the following phenomena: pulse full and very fast; thirst; nausea; frequent vomiting; very severe pain in the left side; fear of dying; bowels constipated since birth; copious lochia, somewhat green mixed with grounds and intolerable on account of the smell; very troubled with strangury.

Inquiry into the nature of her illness. It stems from the retention of the lochia after her first childbearing and from the resulting symptoms; from thick humours not properly

[158] Elizabeth, wife of the Rev. Curwen Hudelstone, vicar of St. Nicholas church. She died, aged 24, after the birth of her second daughter.

evacuated stagnating in the uterus; from the introduction there of a scirrhous tumour with which the uterine vessels were swollen and unable to contract, but discharged all the time a phlegmy material from its orifice which remained open. Afterwards, the urinary viscera were affected by this condition and the putrescence became a permanent state. Moreover, melancholy humours gathered in her abdominal organs and pains like colic arose there. With her second birth, the part of the placenta left behind and the uterus torn by these careless hands are the reason for the symptoms I have noted down. (Perhaps the appearance of the urine arises from an ulcer in the vagina.)

The fever is partly caused by her milk, but symptomatically by the laceration of the uterus and retention of the afterbirth. Her *indisposition, vomiting* and *sickness* come partly from the sympathy of the stomach with the uterus, partly from the copious flow of lochia and its very great stench, and partly from the turgid melancholy humours. The vomit seemed greenish. *Pains* came partly from the laceration of the uterus erosion and its inflammation and partly perhaps from the black bile spread throughout her whole abdomen. The type of lochia was from the afterbirth with ground-laden blood and other humours decaying in the cavity of the uterus and perhaps as a result of this the material of the uterus itself putrefying. The following indications for a cure should hold good. To restrain the gangrene of the uterus by containing the attack of fever and by expelling the putrefying humours from the uterus as quickly as possible, as her strength allows. To collect the melancholy humours in the intestine and to cleanse them gently.

The rise of the fever is halted by the pains easing and her thirst being removed and by diluting or softening the putrid or acrid humours. Putrid humours were expelled from the uterus in a fair quantity with a moderate flow of the lochia. Diet should be from barley or chicken broth and bread saps copiously taken with a little Canary wine late in the day.

Day 5. I prescribed bolus A and draught B to be taken immediately and repeated in the evening.

A. Powdered crabs eyes 1 scruple; Salt of nitre 15 gr; Castor 5 gr; Confection of Kermes berry. Make up a bolus.

B. Black barley water 1 oz; Pennyroyal water 1 oz; Spirit of lavender 20 drops; Oil of sal volatile 20 drops; Liquid laudanum 12 drops; Opium 2 scruples. Make a draught.

This calmed the fever and dulled the pain till the following mid-day, then the pain returned nearly at its previous level, with vomiting of greenish matter and the return of all the rest of the symptoms. For the vomiting, in the morning I had prescribed the former julep and pills with the addition of 5 gr of saffron.

C. Black barley water 3½ oz; Pennyroyal water 3½ oz; Bryony water 1 oz; Spirit of lavender 1 scruple; Oil of sal volatile 1 scruple; Tincture of saffron 1 scruple; Sugar 2½ scruples. Make a julep.

She took one, but on account of the sickness she refused the rest. I prescribed instead an anodyne drink, part to be taken at 5 p.m. and the rest at midnight. With this she was able to get relief from the pain, but she was devastated by sleeplessness and restlessness all night. Meanwhile the flow of lochia grew very great and similar to the variety first described, and her breasts grew hard with milk. Her pulse was slighter and weaker.

Day 6. About mid-day the pain returned very seriously and her stomach was gripped with spasms and she had convulsions, chills, delirium, constant nausea, great discomfort, frequent vomiting, a strong flow of lochia and her flesh came bathed in recurring, stinking sweats mixed with grumous fluids. To ease her stomach I prescribed julep D and to ease the pains, an enema of diluted sugary water and an anodyne draught; by doing this her pains were eased at night, but her lochia continued to flow strongly.

D. Salt of wormwood 1½ scruples; Lemon juice 2 oz; Strong cinnamon water 2 oz; Milk 2 oz; Oil 2 oz; Spirit of lavender 1 scruple; Sugar 2½ scruples. Mix together.

Her delirium lifted from time to time. Profuse cold sweats.

Day 7. In the morning she complained of heartburn, sickness and headaches. Her pulse was really fast and much fainter than before. She took powder E with Canary wine at 11 a.m., then she continued to be vexed with sickness, pain, discomfort and vomiting until 8 or 9 p.m.

E. Crabs eyes 25 gr; American mulberry 5 gr; Sal Prunella 15 gr; Mix together.

F. Cinnamon water 2 oz; Milk 2 oz; Powdered crabs eyes 25 gr; Sal Prunella 20 gr; Liquid laudanum 24 drops; Opium syrup 2 scruples. Make the draught and take half immediately, then the rest after 4 hours and when there is pain and discomfort.

She was not able to take the anodyne draughts I prescribed for her yesterday after the loss of her strength. Her pulse was very weak, very fast and irregular. There was cold in her extremities and cold sweats.

Day 8. About 2 a.m. her spirit departed in peace.

To the most worthy Mr. Cope, M.D., from Wm. Brownrigg. 14th June 1739.

78 Miss Todd, a beautiful girl, well endowed and robust, aged 19.

I have nothing to say about the temperament, age or physical condition of this honest girl whom I am sending to you for consultation, for you will best be able to observe these things when you see her yourself. I wish, however, to say that she was born of normal, healthy parents and is not tainted either with scrofula or any dangerous inherited disease. Indeed, because this well-born girl has been affected by a most persistent illness since she was of tender years and various things may perhaps have slipped her memory, I think it is necessary to describe briefly the history of her illness just as I have heard it, partly from the patient, partly from her mother and partly from my own findings.

When she was about six years old, our patient, after what was wrongly thought to be smallpox, was affected by cacochymia. Next, over a long period of time, she suffered from an intermittent fever which was cured by using Peruvian bark. Finally, at about the age of nine she had pleurisy and this illness went on to a lung abscess. Suddenly, a large quantity of foul pus was coughed up from the abscess which had ruptured. The unhappy girl felt very ill because of the large quantities of sputum she was producing and the slow fever, and she was reduced to a state of great weakness. Finally, a swelling appeared in her right side, which, when she was about eleven, was opened using caustics. From time to time purulent material was discharged. Her cough and other consumptive symptoms disappeared, she put on weight and felt well in other respects except that a scar formed at the orifice of the abscess. Some retained pus found its way to a nearby site by another route, from which it occasionally discharged.

After drinking fermented liquors, her upper right arm was affected by a sensation of cold and very severe pain, then the affected side became moderately inflamed and whenever her whole chest was flushed with an erysipeloid redness her breathing became difficult, and the ribs on the right side were drawn up as it were by a cord from the inside. These symptoms were present until the fistula was incised and one or two little drops of pus were discharged, then all her pain stopped for a short while and the orifice of the fistula skinned over again.

The same symptoms continued to recur during each menstrual period. The patient also often noticed that she suffered when she grew warm with exercise or when she caught cold. Sometimes pure blood was discharged, sometimes thin serum. The patient moreover feels in addition to the sensation of heat, a taste in her mouth like that formerly produced by the material she had brought up from the abscess. Once I had learned all these things, and as the young lady did not want to allow a surgeon to examine the affected area, I myself prepared to examine the same part at close quarters. First of all, I observed that the orifice of the fistula was very small. I therefore prepared a fine lead speculum which I introduced through the orifice to the depth of the length of my thumb beside the sternum, bending it downwards slightly toward the place where the abscess had originally been incised; indeed I was unable to introduce the instrument by any other route. Then, using a syphon which I had ready to hand, I injected a very small quantity of warm mercury round about, then I tried pressing the sides of the orifice in all directions but I could not express one drop of the liquid I had injected. This, however, was returned the following night, now mixed with pus.

So, from this case history which I have recounted, it can be deduced that at the time the patient was suffering from pleurisy and peripneumonia. The lungs and pleura became adherent to each other and this was undoubtedly where the abscess formed later. The purulent material gradually eroded the lungs and pleura and so formed an abscess near the external wall of the thorax. When the abscess sealed itself off prematurely, the contents found another way out, perhaps through the lung and having penetrated into the very cavity of the chest through the fistula, which was a patent channel inside the chest, they were discharged. Whether this material is contained in a sinus or whether it flows freely through the whole thoracic cavity I do not fully understand; however, for many reasons I favour the first means.

Very similar cases to this one are mentioned throughout the literature:
"There is a memorable case history in Willis's *Pharmaceut. Rational.* part 2, para. 1, chapter II[159]—on abscesses. It is about a nobleman who had a huge abscess which ruptured and he brought up a large quantity of thick, foul-smelling, purulent material every day until he was reduced to a state of marasmus. When the abscess had tracked from the left side of the sternum to between the 5th and 6th vertebrae, the offensive sputum entirely cleared up within a fortnight. The opening in his side changed to a discharging sinus, through which copious fluid was discharged every day for eighteenth months, and

[159] Willis, *Pharmaceutice rationalis*, 1677. There is an similar account of a gentleman in section I, chap. XI, but some of the details are different.

meanwhile the worthy gentleman showed no sign of improvement. Finally, the sinus continued across to his arms and around the breast bone which neither fell prey to this illness nor defended against it."

"Another remarkable case is to be found in T. Bonet, *Sepulchret. Anat.* Book 2, para. 9. Additamenta Obs. 4[160]—about a young man suffering from pleurisy, a condition which was degenerating into an empyema. He was not yet weakened by the effects of pain, and with unimpaired strength; he suffered from a swelling between the 5th and 6th ribs on the right side which opened spontaneously in that place which had been predicted. Once this wound had discharged pus, it tended to close up, and after this the patient followed his usual occupation in due manner, and he observed nothing abnormal in his chest, no difficulty in breathing and no pus in his sputum, until exactly one year later when his fistula reappeared, caused by a paracentesis. This new empyema, discharging more or less oily material, seemed to originate from that same opening as the one which discharged the contents of his discharging sinus previously. This fistula or sinus discharged pus, sometimes in the mornings, at others in the evenings. He died, after continuing his usual occupation for five years whenever his fistula allowed, and the fistula was not to blame for his death. About a year before he died he developed dropsy because of great dietary bouts, and particularly on account of a drinking contest. At post mortem, all the abdominal regions were found to be healthy, but the right lung was destroyed, while the left one was intact."

See below—Abstract of a case from the Edinburgh *Medical Essays*[161] [later insertion in English].

"I myself have known quite a few patients who had a silvery thoracic fistula for 25 or 30 years, and who led perfectly normal lives. There is a passage in Aquapendente, *Chirurgica* Book 5, chapter 46 about thoracic fistula—see Paré book 9, chapter 31, and in the same work he described 'those which for some reason are the most difficult to cure'."

[Latin]

Having considered all these matters carefully, I have thought it necessary to dilate the orifice of the fistula and to keep it continually open so that it is like a trickling spring. By this means one can prevent the distension and erosion of the sinus by the material retained within it. In order to implement this policy adequately, it is necessary to promote good diet and good digestion and to aid beneficial secretions and excretions by using the following pills on a long-term basis.

> Electuary of myrrh ½ oz; Liquorice extract ½ oz; Saffron 2 oz; Strasbourg turpentine. Make a pill weighing 5 gr and take 2 together in the morning and at night. Drink milk with the above.

The diet should be light and not at all spicy, consisting of milk, farinaceous foods, tender meat and easily digestible fish. Peppery, smoked, dried and salted foods are to be avoided,

[160] Bonet, *Sepulchretum sive anatomia practica*, 1700, vol. 1, bk II, section VI, p. 674.
[161] The source of this quotation has not been identified.

also fibrous vegetables. Drinks should be just of pure water. Exercise and physical work must be moderate. All violent exertion should be avoided. Emotional upsets should be prudently restrained.

Also to be avoided is studying at night. The patient should rise to greet the rising sun. Adequate clothing should cover the body. During menstrual periods footbaths are beneficial. These matters are now being judged by very experienced physicians. This well-connected young lady is in good health in other respects and attends to her duties energetically. I hardly think I should use more violent medications which might subject her to the risk of becoming worse.

So—should the fistula be emptied completely by making other incisions at a lower level? Or should it be kept open with a silver cannula rather than a wick? Or would it be better to withdraw the pus from the sinus by other channels to other areas? I should very much like to know from more experienced doctors what other measures should be carried out in the future and I humbly subject the measures I have already taken to the judgement of these same physicians.
Given under my hand 18th May, 1739.

[The remaining notes have been inserted in English.]

Dr. Edward Barry of Cork mentions a case in the *Medical Essays*, Vol. 1, Obs. XXVI,[162] of a soldier seized with a Peripneumony which terminated in an abscess of the lungs on the right side, which being broke discharged a fetid pus; by lying on the opposite side the quantity discharged was increased. His body was much emaciated by frequent colliquative dejections attended with perpetual nausea, so that he died about twelve weeks after he was first seized. We found a strong adhesion of his lungs to the pleura on the right side where he had frequent pain & to the diaphragm. Examining into the purulent cavity, we found it continued through the diaphragm about an inch deep into the gibous part of the liver which closely adhered to the diaphragm: the length of this sinus was about six inches and its diameter in the liver was about three, but more narrow in the lungs. The rest of the lobe of the lungs was entirely sound.

A case published in the *Ph. Trans*. No. 285 by Dr. Wright. See Abridg. Vol. II, Part II, Pag. 26.[163]

Mrs. Jane Terry aged 18 of a fresh complexion and pritty fleshy was in May 1701 seized with the smallpox of a favourable distinct kind but attended with a little difficulty of breathing which gradually increased till about the 7th day from the first appearance of the smallpox she began to spit Blood which was raised up by a Cough, in three or four days time twas changed into a very viscuous Phlegm as red as blood, of a very strong smell, of which she would discharge above a pint in twenty four hours. By degrees she recovered again and continued very well from July till near Christmass. Three weeks before Christmas she perceived herself affected with a shortness of Breath, & a fullness and

[162] *Medical essays and observations*, 1733, pp. 273–4.

[163] *The Philosophical Transactions from the year 1700 to 1720*, Abridg'd, Part II, London, B. Motte, 1721, vol. 23, number 285, 1703, pp. 1372–85.

weight in her left side, & when she turned in Bed from the left side to the right, she felt as if a weight fell from the left to the right side, and made her breath short and cough. These Complaints increased daily till Christmass, when she began to spit up a considerable quantity of fluid and digested Pus, oftimes very stinking and offensive. She only coughed at intervalls when she perceived something of a fullness in her Breast, and then could not cease coughing until she had brought up two or three spoonfulls or more of the fetid Pus. This she did chiefly at morning, Afternoon & at Night. D^r^. Wright advised her to lye often upon the Bed with her Head reaching down to the chamber floor, leaning upon her left arm. In this Posture she could at any time set the Pus a running out of her Mouth, until the whole quantity then collected in her Breast was discharged, & then she would get up and seemed perfectly well, untill the Cough again returned after the shortness of Breath.

The Expectoration often abated, but was again increased upon any little Cold, and in this way she continued till the beginning of May, being all that time free from a fever and having her Menses regularly, and eating and sleeping pritty well. About the beginning of May she was seized with a Chillness one afternoon, and then grew feverish, then a rash appeared which went off in about fourteen days, but left her in a Hectick with redness of her Cheeks towards Evening, Night Sweats, continual Looseness, extream wasting of her flesh and at length a swelling in her Legs though she kept her bed. The day after the rash appeared, D^rs^. Walker, Forlesse & Pitts in Consultation concluded that there was an Viscous Ulcer in her lungs and an adhesion of the Lungs to her left side which they judged from the foregoing signs and from some little Pain she felt in her side in discharging the Pus. They also unanimously agreed that an Apertion to her Side was necessary. From some little knotts which they felt betwixt the 7th & 8th Ribs sursum numerando, & from some other Circumstances unrelated, they judged that the Lungs adhered in that part but for fear that the Caustick should spread to the Glands of the Breast they thought it more proper to apply it between the 6th & 7th Ribs, which was accordingly done by M^r^. Cowper as soon as he could he took it off & with his knife passed gently into the cavity of the Breast, whence issued a bloodish Water but no Pus, by bending his Probe he found the Adhesion reach to the lower edge of the 7th rib, before the Iscar was separated the Pus began to flow at every dressing, the Matter or Pus which flowed from her side, had an intolerable offensive Stench & tarnished the end of the silver probe wch was passed into the Cavity of the Abscess. the Lungs wch touched by the Probe, did not afford any sensation, but if the Heart was touched by the finger she grew much disordered, pale and ready to faint. M^r^. Cowper makes no doubt that the pus came from the Abscess, the bitterish Taste of Myrrh w^h^. injected coming into her Mouth as soon as she was affected by the fever she ceased to spit, & afterwards the Pus was only discharged by the knife. By August she was cured, her side being healed up, and in October the Catamenia returned, wch had stopt in May.[164]

[164] A case of lung abscess recorded in great detail. It gives a fascinating insight into Brownrigg's persistence in trying to find the best method of relieving his patient's symptoms, and his willingness to seek a second opinion, but, to add a somewhat cynical note, Miss Todd was from a respectable, well-off family who would have paid him well.

[The following pages were all written in English and have here been reproduced exactly, with all the eccentricities of spelling and punctuation.]

GENERAL OBSERVATIONS

Abstracted from a Book entitled A view of the present Evidence for and against Mrs. Stephens Medicines as a solvent for the Stone, containing 155 Cases with some Experiments and Observations, by David Hartley a Physician 1739.[165]

In these Cases are first enumerated all the Phenomena which appeared before the use of the Medicines, viz. Nephritick pains, and other signs of Stones in the Kidnies or Ureters often preceeding diagnostick signs of the Stone in the Bladder; passing of gravel Stones by the Penis. Difficulty of Urine, most acute pains, sharpness and scalding in making of Urine, oftimes a stoppage relieved by standing on the Crown of the Head or else a Suppression of Urine for several days; sometimes an incontinence of Urine, Pains in the Penis especially the Glans; violent strainings and motion to make Water; a frequent Tenismus; a sensation of weight and pressure at the neck of the Bladder, and a perception of the Stones changing its place upon altering the Posture of the Body; cruel grevious and almost intolerable pains in the urinary Vessels much increased by motion; Urine sometimes fetid, frequently bloody, or mixt with grumous blood after motion, or constantly of a Coffee colour, sometimes clear, often depositing a thick Mucous gelatinous heavy sediment. In many afflicted with these Symptomes the Stones had been found by Mr. Cheselden, Mr. Fern, Hawkins and other skillfull Surgeons, by the Catheter. And in others several other large stones had been felt at one time in the Bladder by introducing the Finger into the Anus. Many of these Patients had been afflicted with these symptoms for several years and were upwards of seventy years old, and at the same time laboured under other Illnesses, and were generally weak and infirm and had a bad Habit of Body from the violence of the Symptoms, yet have been perfectly releived and entirely cured of all the foregoing Complaints by a long and constant use of Mrs. Stephens's Medicines.

The Medicines do increase the straining and motion to make Water, and at first do generally occasion the Pains to be more sore and cruel than usual, oftimes increasing them untill they are almost intolerable. These violent racking pains continue a longer or shorter time according to the difference of Constitution magnitude figure or Hardness of the Stone and other Circumstances. The pains do still continue very acute while any of the calcalouse Substance is said to remain, but do generally abate about the time at which it is thought the Stone begins to break; which in some had happened in three or four days, but most commonly it is three or four weeks; in others not before the Remedies have been taken for a quarter of a year; and some who certainly had the Stone in the Bladder have used them constantly for sixteen Months together without receiving any Benefit. But oftimes great and ponderous Stones have been broken or discharged from the Bladder by a years Course of the Medicines, altho such Patients have frequently afterwards remained subject to Nephritic Ailments. Also after a years constant use of the Medicines, when the Stones in the Bladder were thought to have been dissolved, there have still remained

[165] David Hartley, *A view of the present evidence for and against Mrs. Stephens's Medicines*, London, S. Harding, 1739.

stones in the Kidnies; for (as a learned Gent: observes in his own case) altho from a great many instances we may conclude that they produce the same Effect in the Kidnies as in the Bladder, yet it does not happen so soon because that in the latter the medicated urine stays a long while with the Stone, where as in the former it only drops in small quantities on the Stone in its Passage. He might also have added other powerfull Argument viz: That in the Kidnies the stone lyes at rest and therefore wants that constant Attrition, occasioned by the motion of the Stone in the Bladder, and the continual pressure of the Bladder upon it on all Sides, whereby such parts as only adhere loosely to the Stone will be continually wearing away and rubbing off. But tho for these reasons, the Medicines are not so well fitted to dissolve Stones in the Kidnies as in the Bladder, yet from many observations we may conclude that they are exceeding efficacious in forcing away and expelling gravel Stones lodged in the Kidnies, which are not too large to pass.

When the Stone is supposed to be acted upon by the medicated Urine in such a manner as to disunite its parts, which is called dissolving the Stone, then there commonly appears voided with the Urine Bits or Flakes of white stoney matter in a soft state, yeilding to a light pressure and crumbling between the fingers, and hardning again when exposed sometime in the Air, these Flakes are of various magnitudes some being so large as to occasion great pain and trouble in passing; several Gentlemen upon comparing together the flakes which they passed have found them exactly alike. They have sometimes had a hollow side as if they were crusts of a larger Stone, and sometimes pieces have been voided consisting of several Coats to six in number. Sixty six flakes of different sizes have been discharged in 24 hours. Sometimes large fragments of stone have been voided with great pain being partly white and soft, partly hard and brown. Others have compared what they discharged to Ashes, scaly Matter, flakes like salt hard and sharp, coarse gravel, Gritt, rotten Stone, chalky matter slaking like lime, rotten egg Shells, porus shells of stone. These substances have ceased coming for several weeks, whilst signs of the Stone remaining, but have again begun to be discharged, the inward substance of the Stone in such cases being judged to be harder than some of the outer Coats. After these substances have been long discharged, at length a stone has often come away, and then all the pain and trouble has ceased. These stones have oft appeared spungy, whitish and uneaven, and soft as if acted upon by a menstruum; and are supposed to be the Kernels of larger stones. Whilst these stoney flakes are passed the urine is sometimes turbid and in others quite clear. Many have been relieved by the Medicines without discharging any flakes, their urine being then observed to have a white heavy Sediment judged to be the Stone reduced into impalpable particles. Others have found themselves eased after discharging a reddish slime or mucous Matter or various colours, tho this but rarely happens. Several persons after taking the medicines a short time, have voided large quantities of gravel Stones, which not being too large to pass, are expelled by the force of the Remedies without being much altered, one Gentleman voided 55 of these Stones in two days, some being as large as a rouncivel pea, others no bigger than a pin head. When all these flakes or other calculous concretions are come away, the patients (not withstanding the use of the Remedies) do then become perfectly easy and free from their pains and other complaints, and so have continued for several years after they have returned to their wonted Exercises, occupations, and ways of living.

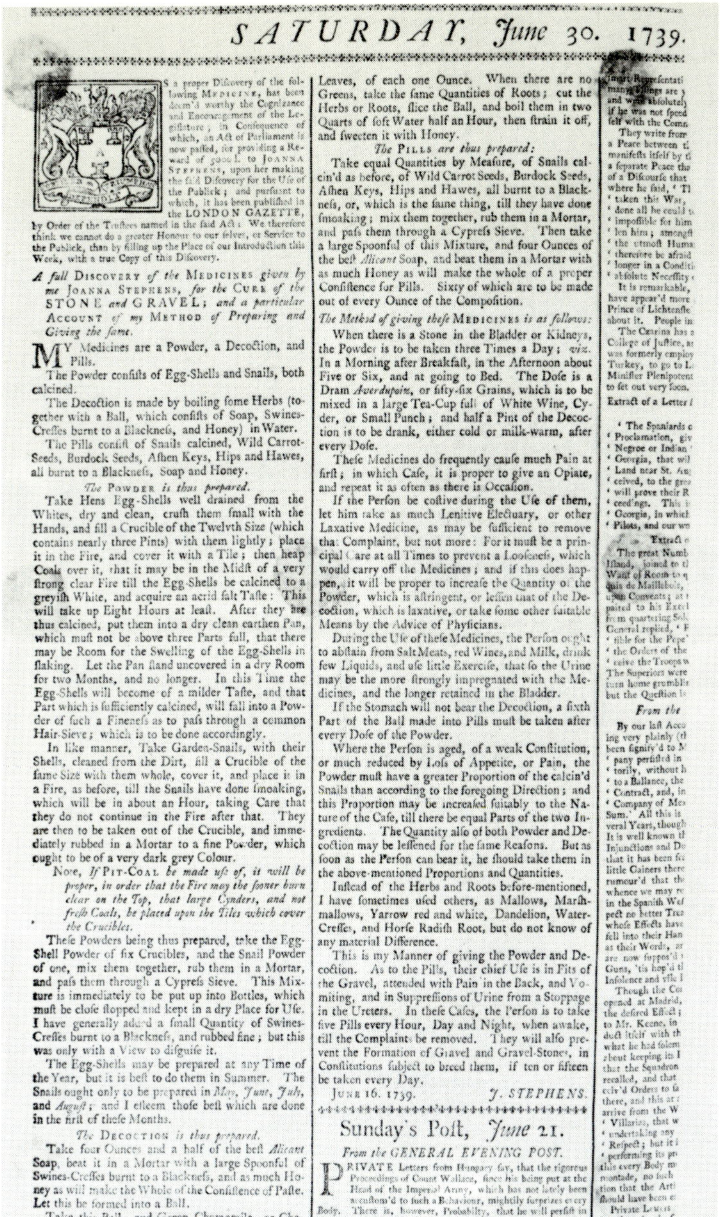

SATURDAY, June 30. 1739.

As a proper Discovery of the following Medicine, has been deem'd worthy the Cognizance and Encouragement of the Legislature; in Consequence of which, an Act of Parliament is now passed, for providing a Reward of 5000 l. to Joanna Stephens, upon her making the said Discovery for the Use of the Publick; and pursuant to which, it has been published in the LONDON GAZETTE, by Order of the Trustees named in the said Act: We therefore think we cannot do a greater Honour to our selves, or Service to the Publick, than by filling up the Place of our Introduction this Week, with a true Copy of this Discovery.

A full Discovery *of the* Medicines *given by me* Joanna Stephens, *for the* Cure *of the* STONE *and* GRAVEL; *and a particular* Account *of my* Method *of Preparing and Giving the same.*

My Medicines are a Powder, a Decoction, and Pills.

The Powder consists of Egg-Shells and Snails, both calcined.

The Decoction is made by boiling some Herbs (together with a Ball, which consists of Soap, Swines-Cresses burnt to a Blackness, and Honey) in Water.

The Pills consist of Snails calcined, Wild Carrot-Seeds, Burdock Seeds, Ashen Keys, Hips and Hawes, all burnt to a Blackness, Soap and Honey.

The Powder *is thus prepared.*

Take Hens Egg-Shells well drained from the Whites, dry and clean, crush them small with the Hands, and fill a Crucible of the Twelvth Size (which contains nearly three Pints) with them lightly; place it in the Fire, and cover it with a Tile; then heap Coals over it, that it may be in the Midst of a very strong clear Fire till the Egg-Shells be calcined to a greyish White, and acquire an acrid salt Taste: This will take up Eight Hours at least. After they are thus calcined, put them into a dry clean earthen Pan, which must not be above three Parts full, that there may be Room for the Swelling of the Egg-Shells in flaking. Let the Pan stand uncovered in a dry Room for two Months, and no longer. In this Time the Egg-Shells will become of a milder Taste, and that Part which is sufficiently calcined, will fall into a Powder of such a Fineness as to pass through a common Hair-Sieve; which is to be done accordingly.

In like manner, Take Garden-Snails, with their Shells, cleaned from the Dirt, fill a Crucible of the same Size with them whole, cover it, and place it in a Fire, as before, till the Snails have done smoaking, which will be in about an Hour, taking Care that they do not continue in the Fire after that. They are then to be taken out of the Crucible, and immediately rubbed in a Mortar to a fine Powder, which ought to be of a very dark grey Colour.

Note, *If* Pit-Coal *be made use of, it will be proper, in order that the Fire may the sooner burn clear on the Top, that large Cynders, and not fresh Coals, be placed upon the Tiles which cover the Crucibles.*

These Powders being thus prepared, take the Egg-Shell Powder of six Crucibles, and the Snail Powder of one, mix them together, rub them in a Mortar, and pass them through a Cypress Sieve. This Mixture is immediately to be put up into Bottles, which must be close stopped and kept in a dry Place for Use. I have generally added a small Quantity of Swines-Cresses burnt to a Blackness, and rubbed fine; but this was only with a View to disguise it.

The Egg-Shells may be prepared at any Time of the Year, but it is best to do them in Summer. The Snails ought only to be prepared in *May*, *June*, *July*, and *August*; and I esteem those best which are done in the first of these Months.

The Decoction *is thus prepared.*

Take four Ounces and a half of the best *Alicant* Soap, beat it in a Mortar with a large Spoonful of Swines-Cresses burnt to a Blackness, and as much Honey as will make the Whole of the Consistence of Paste. Let this be formed into a Ball.

Take this Ball, and Green Chamomile, or Chamomile Flowers, Sweet Fennel, Parsley, and Burdock Leaves, of each one Ounce. When there are no Greens, take the same Quantities of Roots; cut the Herbs or Roots, slice the Ball, and boil them in two Quarts of soft Water half an Hour, then strain it off, and sweeten it with Honey.

The Pills *are thus prepared:*

Take equal Quantities by Measure, of Snails calcin'd as before, of Wild Carrot Seeds, Burdock Seeds, Ashen Keys, Hips and Hawes, all burnt to a Blackness, or, which is the same thing, till they have done smoaking; mix them together, rub them in a Mortar, and pass them through a Cypress Sieve. Then take a large Spoonful of this Mixture, and four Ounces of the best *Alicant* Soap, and beat them in a Mortar with as much Honey as will make the whole of a proper Consistence for Pills. Sixty of which are to be made out of every Ounce of the Composition.

The Method of giving these Medicines *is as follows:*

When there is a Stone in the Bladder or Kidneys, the Powder is to be taken three Times a Day; *viz.* In a Morning after Breakfast, in the Afternoon about Five or Six, and at going to Bed. The Dose is a Dram *Averdupois*, or fifty-six Grains, which is to be mixed in a large Tea-Cup full of White Wine, Cyder, or Small Punch; and half a Pint of the Decoction is to be drank, either cold or milk-warm, after every Dose.

These Medicines do frequently cause much Pain at first; in which Case, it is proper to give an Opiate, and repeat it as often as there is Occasion.

If the Person be costive during the Use of them, let him take as much Lenitive Electuary, or other Laxative Medicine, as may be sufficient to remove that Complaint, but not more: For it must be a principal Care at all Times to prevent a Looseness, which would carry off the Medicines; and if this does happen, it will be proper to increase the Quantity of the Powder, which is astringent, or lessen that of the Decoction, which is laxative, or take some other suitable Means by the Advice of Physicians.

During the Use of these Medicines, the Person ought to abstain from Salt Meats, red Wines, and Milk, drink few Liquids, and use little Exercise, that so the Urine may be the more strongly impregnated with the Medicines, and the longer retained in the Bladder.

If the Stomach will not bear the Decoction, a sixth Part of the Ball made into Pills must be taken after every Dose of the Powder.

Where the Person is aged, of a weak Constitution, or much reduced by Loss of Appetite, or Pain, the Powder must have a greater Proportion of the calcin'd Snails than according to the foregoing Direction; and this Proportion may be increased suitably to the Nature of the Case, till there be equal Parts of the two Ingredients. The Quantity also of both Powder and Decoction may be lessened for the same Reasons. But as soon as the Person can bear it, he should take them in the above-mentioned Proportions and Quantities.

Instead of the Herbs and Roots before-mentioned, I have sometimes used others, as Mallows, Marshmallows, Yarrow red and white, Dandelion, Water-Cresses, and Horse Radish Root, but do not know of any material Difference.

This is my Manner of giving the Powder and Decoction. As to the Pills, their chief Use is in Fits of the Gravel, attended with Pain in the Back, and Vomiting, and in Suppressions of Urine from a Stoppage in the Ureters. In these Cases, the Person is to take five Pills every Hour, Day and Night, when awake, till the Complaint be removed. They will also prevent the Formation of Gravel and Gravel-Stones, in Constitutions subject to breed them, if ten or fifteen be taken every Day.

June 16. 1739. *J. STEPHENS.*

Sunday's Post, *June* 21.

From the GENERAL EVENING POST.

PRIVATE Letters from Hungary say, that the rigorous Proceedings of Count Wallace, since his being put at the Head of the Imperial Army, which has not lately been accustom'd to such a Behaviour, mightily surprizes every Body. There is, however, Probability, that he will persist in this Sort of Conduct, having determined, at any Rate, to establish good Order and Discipline in the Army. He has made

Plate 4: This page has been pasted into the Casebook as an introduction to a lengthy consideration of "The Stone". It was published as a supplement to the *Newcastle Courant* on Saturday June 30th, 1739, and as there were no newspapers published in Whitehaven at that time, it may be conjectured that Brownrigg may have taken this as his regular paper. Allowing for the state of road transport, he would not have received it until later in July.

In the *Gentleman's Magazine* for April, 1738, the advertisement appeared as follows: "Mrs. Stephens has proposed to make her Medicine public on Consideration of £5,000. to be raised by contribution". Joanna Stephens appealed in various other papers and journals, and money began to accumulate. Only a third of the sum was raised from contributors such as the Bishop of Oxford, the Earl of Pembroke, the Duke of Richmond and the Bishop of Gloucester, but as Mrs. Stephens had many influential friends, they applied to Parliament to grant the remaining sum to her, in order to allow it to be made public. Parliament obliged!

The remedy first appeared in the *London Gazette* of June 19th, 1737 and is identical to the insertion in the *Courant*.

SOME INSTANCES. THESE MEDICINES, SOMETIMES UNSUCCESSFULL OR PREJUDICIAL

The use of these Medicines hath not been attended with the desired effects in many for want of Patient and proper Resolution. One Gentleman as was before observed took them sixteen month very regularly without receiving any Benefit.

A Gentleman aged 75 was sounded and a stone found, on o.ber the 8th. he began to take the Medicines, he discharged flakes as in others, but grew feverish and died on Jan:20. after being opened a stone weighing nearly 2 oz was taken out of his Bladder. Mr. Hawkins and Dr. Shaw both testified that it was white on the outside, soft and unequally covered with a cretaceous wch broke of wth great ease like those before voided as appeared by comparing them; the inner part was reddish and harder, so that to an indifferent person it appeared as acted upon by a solvent.

A Gentleman aged 74 takes the Medicines, the Stone in the Bladder is broke but he afterwards died of an Ischury, from Stones in the Kidnies or Ureters. Another voids ulcerous stinking matter for nine years, being also afflicted with the stone, took the remedies for a year but finding no relief discontinued them for a month and then died. In the Bladder were found four smooth Stones as big as Chestnuts, a spongy Stone in the right Kidney and an Ulcer in the left.

DR. HARTLEY'S EXP. ON THE MEDICINES

A clergyman after a wrench in the side, soon after had violent pains which he took for the gravel. He therefore took the Medicines some time and voided a fleshy substance 1½ inch long, and he died being much wasted in a month: Two others affirm that the Medicines occasioned a swelling in their Body and Legs which went off after leaving off taking. Whilst he took the medicines his Urine had a more urinous Smell than usual; was turbid at time of making and alcaline, that is turned Syrup of Violets green and fermented with various kinds of Acids. As far as he could judge the Case is the same with all who take the Medicines. He has lately been informed that common Urine after putrefaction will dissolve and take up the calcalous Incrustations upon the sides and bottoms of Chamber pots. The Medicated Urine does not occasion an incrustation to the sides of the Chamber-pot, but rather dissolves those made by the other Urine. It appears from the Exp: of Mons. Littre in the Memoirs de l'Academie Royale and from these of Dr. Hales in his Haemastatics that common Water of several sorts is able to dissolve a Variety of Stones from the humane Body. This shows that an acrimonious Menstruum is not necessary for that purpose, and that the mere aqueousness of Urine may perhaps have a dissolving Efficacy, if its concreting incrusting quality could first be destroyed.

The putrid Smell and alcaline quality of the Urine of those that take Mrs. Stephens's Medicines make it probable that this concreting incrusting quality is actually destroyed in it, and favour its dissolving power. For putrefaction is one kind of dissolution and is very apt to propagate itself in contiguous Bodies; and alcaline salts are powerfull Solvents. Since also urine in becoming Vinegar takes up its own Tartar, and the Mineral Waters in putrefying take up their own Incrustations or Tartars, as Dr. Hales assured me; it seems probable from Analogy that putrial Urine should also dissolve its Tartar; that is the Gravel and Stones generated in it.

Dr. Hartley also made several accurate and laborious Experiments by digesting Stones and pieces of the same Stone of the Human Bladder with a gentle Heat equal to that of the

Urine in the Bladder, in four different Liquors viz. New River Water, New River Water with Mrs. Stephens's Powder, Common Urine and His own Alcaline Urine. He does not mention his having put fresh common Urine as the other became alcaline, but says that as each liquour evaporated he filled the vessel up with fresh of the same kind. He observed that from time to time those in the Hide Park Water, Hide Park Water and Powder and in the Medicated Alcaline Urine, had a whiteness in their surface, wch when it was rubbed off left the Stone of its natural colour, but in those most affected white Scales fell off upon being rubbed and some of them were corroded and honey combed. And one in the Medicated Urine was cracked in several places. He oftimes rubbed off the loose matter from their Surfaces, and rubbed the Stones in common urine also, after several Months digestion the Stones in the above mentioned liquours became so small that he ceased rubbing them, at length they were intirely dissolved those in the Medicated Urine in the shortest time, next those in New River Water, then those in N. River Water with ye Powder. After all these were dissolved the Stones were taken out of the common Urine, and being carefully rubbed were found to be increased in weight by several additional Incrustations.

CONCLUSIONS DRAWN FROM THE CASES & EXP: BY D. HARTLEY

1. Mrs. Stephens's Medicines must in general be innocent and safe. For a large number have taken them in great quantities and for a long time yet few seem to have received any Injury.

2. These Medicines have done great Service in the Stone and gravel. It has not been proper to publish the neglects, irregularities, and infirmities of particular persons, therefore great allowances ought to be given on those accounts. If they were under the direction of Physicians, and the Patients themselves constant in taking them, and regular in other particulars, more good might be done by them.

3. These Medicines do not make the flakes and fragments voided by those that take them. It appears from the foregoing Exp: that the medicated alcaline urine has no such incrusting concreting power. If the medicines made the flakes and fragments, these would continue to come away as long as the medicines were taken; but the contrary of this appears from the cases. The form of many of the flakes shows that they must have been separated from the Surface of a stone.

   But the previous incrustation and subsequent Separation are of a nature so contrary to each other, that one does not know how to reconcile them.

4. The Cases of those that take the Medicines cannot be accounted for, from accident. For there are no accidental Instances where persons first void white rotten Scales and fragments, in the Quantity and Variety mentioned in the Cases, then intire Stones or large solid Pieces and lastly grow free from their complaints: or allowing that this did happen once in a thousand times still it would not account for the large number of extrordinary Cases here published.

5. The Urine of those that take these Medicines, has a stone dissolving power. This appears partly from the Exp: but is clearly proved from all the Facts taken together, it being impossible to account for them upon any other Suppositione.

From what hath been said we may judge what digree of Credit ought to be given to the following objections, published in the Magasines.

A Stone of the Bladder being put into a mixture of New River Water and the powder, a white soft substance was observed upon its surface, the stone being taken out and suffered to dry without having been rubbed was found to be increased in weight.

From wch Exp: a stone—generating rather than a dissolving power is argued in the Medicines. This is endeavoured to be proved from Dr. Hartleys own Case, who was examined with the Catheter before he began the use of the Medicines and no Stone found; but being examined again after he had taken the Medicines some time a Stone was found.

The Powder infused in water with a little corrosive sublimate gave a yellow colour. The powder and Ball being mixt together made a strong escharotic, whence it was concluded that the powder was Calx viva slaked in the Air wch being mixed with 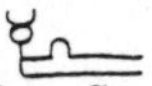 and the Ball produced exactly the same Effects; The Ball Was allowed by Mrs. Stephens herself to be mostly soap. Both the powder and Ball were conjectured to be made black with Charcoal.

It was therefore argued that such caustick corrosive mixtures must be highly pernicious when received in to the Body and was so far from being a solvent that it was a generater of the Stone.

Mr. Sharp in his Treatise on Surgical operations published in 1739 says, that those uneasy sensations and violent pains which torment those afflicted with the Stone, do proceed from an Inflamation of the Coats of the Bladder, and that in order to produce them a particular disposition of Body is necessary as well as the presence of the Stone for the Stone itself frequently gives no pain and people will have long intervalls of ease altho the Stone remains in the Bladder. That therefore such Remedies as will prevent that Inflamatory Diathesis of the Bladder will also palliate the pains and that for this purpose nothing is equal to a Milk Diet with Honey. He further takes notice that the Ease frequently given by palliative Remedies of this kind hath made many believe in several ages that they had discovered remedies which would dissolve the stone, altho no safe Remedy hath yet been found which will produce this Effect.

NB: It is hardly credible that diuretick irritating medicines which increase the pains when first used, should afterwards palliate and ease them.

NATURE, EFFECTS & MANNER OF OPERATION OF MRS. STEPHENS' MEDICINES[166]

Nature of the Powder.

The Powder is an Alcaline Calx. wch would make a strong Cement and hath some sulphureous particles remaining mixed with it as appears from its Colour. By being so long exposed to the Air in slaking it imbibes great plenty of acid aereal particles which being united to the alcaline Calx do constitute an alcaline Sal Murarium or Calcarium.

[166] Brownrigg's own observations.

OPERATION & EFFECTS OF THE POWDER

The powder is a strong diuretick, having when taken alone brought away Stones and gravelly Matter in large quantities. It is also powerfully detergent having cleansed the Ureters and Kidnies from mucous matter there lodged. It is very drying and occasions costiveness. It may be given to advantage even in Ulcers of the Kidnies. It also cures Incontinence of Urine. In a certain person who laboured under difficulty of the Stone, they seem to have occasioned an Ischary by irritating and inflaming the Neck of the Bladder. Some have taken them alone for the Stone a long time together without receiving any Benefit.

NATURE & OPERATION OF THE BALLS

Dr. Hartley gives no instances where the Balls have been taken alone altho greater Benefit might be expected from them than from the Powder.

WHICH EFFECTS MAY RESULT FROM THE MIXTURE OF THE POWDER WITH THE BALLS

EFFECTS OF BOTH THE MEDICINES

These medicines w^{n} taken together are exceeding forcing, strongly irritating, stimulating and diuretic. They burn the Urinous salts from a neutral to an alcaline nature which hath not been observed upon the use of any other Remedies. Or perhaps these alcaline salts may be the Salts of the Remedies themselves separated from the mass of Blood by the Kidnies. Whichsoever Case obtains these salts whilst they flow in the Mass of fluids must dissolve its texture and dispose it to putrefaction. Tis a wonder therefore that no one observes these remedies to occasion Thirst or to produce of feverish Heat of Body. Tis also probable that they frequently may occasion inflamations in the Urinary Organs, by their irritating and stimulating qualities, and may dispose these parts to mortify by their putrid nature. Tis probable also that they relax and widen the Urinary passages as well as stimulate, since they oftimes bring away Stones which would not pass before; altho the Patients had had violent strainings and forcings from the irritation. The Medicated alcaline Urine produced by the Use of the Medicines both soften and break the stone in the Bladder and destroy the cohesion subsisting between its parts, but doth not intirely dissolve the Stone as a body is said to be dissolved in a chemical Menstruum. And may therefore be called a Lithotriptic more properly than a true Solvent of the stone.

[Small page inserts in Casebook, written in English.]

My Opinions concerning the Nature of y^{r} Disease

From Attentively considering disorder under Mrs. Watson is afflicted.

From the Symptoms with which you Labour, there does not appear any certain signs of a Stone in the Bladder but the violent pains about the region of the Bladder, and obtuse pains in your right Thigh, frequent in---tions to make walking without any stoppage together with a great thickness at your Stomach do pritty plainly discover a small Stone seated in the right Ureter nigh its Insertion into the Bladder, and therefore may well be accounted too fixed to be moved or too large to pass.

Advice

As the disorder hath been of long continuance, and as the Stone must therefore be very fixed, and probably much increased in its bulk, I would therefore be in vain to attempt to expell it into the Bladder whole as it is. All therefore that can be done in such a Case is to endeavour to dissolve it by means of Mrs. Stephens's Medicines which I am convinced from many observations, have proved in many Cases, are a true solvent of the Stone in the Bladder, But that it will not allways produce the same effect upon Stones in the Kidnies or Ureters. I have great reason to fear there being many Instances where small stones have remained undissolved in the Kidnies after the use. However in such Cases tis better to try probable means that have been dissolving in the Bladder. W^{ch} I would therefore recommend her to try, especially As I beleive they will not be prejudicial to her in other respects, but will rather be of great service for her Asthma and not prejudicial upon other Acc^{t}s.

Directions

That they may be taken so as to be likely to do her service 'tis necessary that she should take them constantly and in such quantity as is directed by Mrs. Stephens in the Account wch she published for the Space of two months at least, whether she finds any Benefit from them or not, Observing the Other Directions wch Mrs. Stephens has given in her printed account of them.

Please to communicate this to Mrs. Watson, and if she is resolved to try the Medicines give her such further Directions as you see necessary, and if any difficulty arise from the use of them upon the Notice I shall give her further instructions.

W. B.

[The following three prescriptions (in Latin) are inserted on small pages. The two for William Hicks relate to the gentleman in Case No. 2 who was then suffering from epidemic fever, but he also appeared to suffer from the Stone.]

William Hicks, Esq.

Electuary of powdered rhubarb 1½ oz; Powdered saffron 1½ scruples; Pound together with diuretic pills of Mrs. Stephens: 10 drops of Aniseed oil; Extract of liquorice. (Dissolve in spring water and add thick syrup to the solution to a binding consistency). Add about the same quantity of Strasbourg turpentine to make up a harder mass of the pill, and make 10 pills of a single drachm from it. Take 3 in the day after 4 oz of this warm decoction.
Marshmallow leaves 2 packs; mallow 2 packs; Liquorice root 1½ oz; Venetian soap 1 oz; Juniper berry 2½ scruples; sea holly root 1½ oz.

After repeated convulsions

Mrs. Stephens' powders for the diuretic pills; Rhubarb; Saffron; Extract of oil of aniseed; Strasbourg turpentine. Make up a paste, gently warming the pestle and stirring at the same time. Make 10 pills of 1 drachm each. Take 5. Three daily after 4 oz of this decoction and continue to use them for an hour.
Marshmallow leaf 2 pecks; Mallow 2 pecks; Liquorice root 1 oz; Juniper berry 2½ scruples; Venetian soap; Honey. Mix the soap with warm spring water and boil to make up 2 pts.

Mrs. Carr.

> Powders for Mrs. Stephens' pills 3 scruples; Electuary of powdered myrrh 2 scruples; Saffron 2 scruples; Juniper oil 1 scruple; Strasbourg turpentine. Make up 10 pills, each of 1 drachm. Venetian soap 5 scruples; Best honey 2 oz; Sassafras oil 5 drops measured exactly.
> This is the mixture for the decoction.

[The following section is written in English, again reproduced with eccentric spelling and punctuation.]

REMEDIES FOR THE STONE

The Revd Dr Kirkpatrick a Physician at Belfast gives the following History in his Case published by Dr. Hartley.[167]

Mr. James Steuart a dissenting Minister has had several Stones in his Bladder for six years in the Spring 1737 he drunk the following decoction:

> For the syrup a mixture of Hollyhock and Wild parsley 4 oz gently boiled in 24 or 26 fl. oz of spring water. Strain and add 2 pts of white wine; 1½ oz Honey. Boil this gently for ¼ hour. Take ½ a pint in a single draught.

By continuing the use of this for 3 Months he passed at several times above 100 very large pieces of Stone, many of them the thickness of half a Straw breadth, were broder than the Strawbreadth and some ½ Inch long. The outside was smooth as polished Marble and convex, the inside rough and concave, he passed likewise a great deal of Slime. By laying together the pieces he could find out the Dimensions of one stone. But there were many other pieces when laid together exhibited a quite different shape from the former whence he concluded he must have had at least two stones. He apprehended that the remedy was too rough and so left off, but found himself easier after it than he had been for four years.

He was afterwards informed of a medicated Scots Ale, which had brought away a large Stone in the Bladder in form of a fine Sediment in the Urine, from Mr. Monteeth, Minister of Buay in Galloway in N. Britain. The Composition is this

> Prescription: Flower of Camomile and Seed of Wild Carrot both 2 pecks; Grass root, sea holly, liquefied Anthamantin, sage leaves each 1 drachm. Combine these in oil with thick Scotch Ale and drink 4 oz like and ordinary potion. Dr. Steuart added leaves of wild parsley, feverfew; berries, elderflower; Juniper.

He had used this constantly for a year past, by which he finds great Ease, and observes in his Urine a very large Sediment exactly of the same Colour with the Shells of Stones which he passed. He can walk four or five Miles a day without Bloody Urine, which he could not do for some years before, and hopes that the Stone will be gradually brought away in the Sediment.

Remedies by various authors praising the breaking of the Stone.

A Gent. in Kent found great releif in the Stone from—Juce of Onions of wch he took half

[167] Hartley, *A view of the present evidence . . .*, pp. 150–2.

a pint for a dose every other Morning. he found a larger quantity over-heated him. See Lobb on Dissolvents of ye Stone C XVIII.

A boy at Norwich who was to have been cut for the Stone was cured by Onion Water. A quarter of a pint may be taken twice a day. it must be made of the same strength as it is of when Onions are boiled for Sauce. Ibidem.

ON THE STONE

Abstracts from a Treatise intitled On Dissolvents of the Stone & On Curing the Stone & Gout by Aliment by Theophilus Lobb M.D. & F.R.S.[168]

Chapter I

The Exp. of Mr. Boyle Dr. Grew Dr. Slare & Dr. Hales plainly prove "That the human calculus consists of a very large quantity of air, with a good quantity of a volatile Alcaline Salt, some Oil, & a little Earth or waste residue. p.2. Therefore, is an Alcaline concretion p.7.

"In countries where the Water is not petrifying the Calculus is generated or produced chiefly in Bodies used to drink wine; and among the great Number of persons whom Dr Cyprianus cut for Stone, there were few but wch. were Wine Drinkers" p.5.

Probably in Italy & Spain & where wine is ye common Drink the Stone wd. be more common if there was not something in their Diet wch prevented its increase p.6. Query: if Acidic p.7

[Marginal note:] Lemon juice dissolves various stones.

Exp. 1.2.3.4. Lemon juice partly dissolves, and partly breaks into fragments white marble, gypsum and Portland Stone on boiling in it. The Dissolution of the Stones mentioned seems to be accomplished by the Acid Particles of ye Juice of Lemons destroying the Union wch. was between the Particles of Air, and the other constituent parts of the several Stones. Whence it appears probable that those particles of Air were as Bards of Union to the other constituent parts of the several Stones p.16.

Chapt. II

The probability of dissolving the Stone either in the Kidnies or Bladder by means of things recd. into ye Stomach as Aliment will appear from the following considerations.

Prop. 1 The Constituent parts of ye Stone are Salt, Air, Oil & Earth, the 2 latter in very inconsiderable quantities in respect of the 2 former.

Prop. 2 These constituent parts exist in all human bodies.

3 and are too abundant in persons afflicted wth. ye Stone & Gout.

Prop. 5 These constituent parts proceed from the Aliment.

Prop. 6 Alcaline & Alcalescent Aliments communicate a petrefying Quality to the Urine. N.B. Amongst these he ranks even spontaneous ascescents or Wines.

Prop. 7 As the Stone is produced & increased by Alcalescents it is reasonable to think it may be diminished in bulk or gradually dissolved by things of a contrary quality received in the Stomach for

1. the Urine may receive qualities from things taken into the Stomach.

[168] Theophilus Lobb, *On dissolvents of the stone . . .*, London, J. Buckland, 1739.

2. That a quality of Dissolvement of the Stone may be communicated to the Urine.

3. There are divers Vegetables used in Aliment wch. will dissolve the Stone out of the Bladder.

A dissolving Quality may be imparted to the Urine as easily as petryfying quality.

Chap. iii.

Continuing Exp. made on the Calculi with Juice of Lemons.

Exp. i July 27, 1738. A fragment of a Calculus weighing 10 grams was put into 2 oz of Lemon Juice and 1 oz of Honey: Aug 5. The Calculus was risen from the Bottom and swam on the Surface of the Liquor. Aug. 7. the Calculus was dissolved into 3 parts. Aug. 24. The 3 divided parts retained their form & appearance but were as soft as Jelly. The Calculus was 28 days in the Liquid.

Exp. Second. A calculus 4 grams being digested in 2 oz of common Punch for 28 days became soft & by gently pressing it between the fingers broke into pieces.

Exp. iii A calculus 14 grams digested in 3 oz Punch for 62 days was easily divided into rough pieces.

Exp. iv A 10 gram calculus and 2 oz Lemon juice digested 24 days the Stone retained its figure but became soft & a Lump of Jelly or thick pap and has nothing in it.

Exp. V A 7 gram calculus being digested 84 days in 2 oz of Lemon Juice remained hard but rub'd pretty easily into a fine powder and being digested 5 hours warm with ye same juice easily pressed into powder.

Exp. Vi A 16 oz calculus was digested 2 Months with 3 oz of Lemon juice, then again 23 days in 3 oz of fresh Juice in all 83 days, it was not dissolved into a soft substance, but with a gentle pressure between the finger was reduced into a gritty matter like large sand.

Exp. Vii Another 8 gram fragment digested 9 days 2 oz of Lemon juice was dissolved into a soft Pap or Jelly.

Exp. Viii A 1 oz 6 gram calculus being digested in 3 oz Lemon juice for 23 days, its outer layer separated easily and the whole was much softened. In all the Digestions no Air Bubbles were produced.

Chapt. IV. Exp. IX. A 7gr calculus and 1½ oz of juice of Rue. being digested 29 days, the stone remained as hard as ever but was burned black

Exp. Xi 3 gr. calculus Turnip juice 4 oz in 23 days, every part of the Stone was dissolved into Jelly.

Exp. XiV 1 gr calculus 2 oz Cyder digested 23 days, the Stone became soft and dissolved.

Exp. XV 12 gr calculus 2 oz of Codlins (apple) juice digested 23 days, the Stone felt soft like wet Clay was divided into parts deminished much in bulk, and easily mashd by pressing.

Chapt. V

In this Chapt. he gives various Exp. made on Calculi with Juce of Mulberries by itself also mist with Water, Brandy & Mulberry Wine. the event was much ye same as in the Exp. made with Juce of Lemons some stones being dissolved into a pap, others breaking into powders, and others remaining hard. Only the dissolving quality seemed rather Stronger in the juce of Mulberries than in Juce of Lemon.

Chap. Vi

Juces of Strawberries, Elderberries, Burgamy Pears & Grapes act upon the Stone much in the same manner with Juce of Mulberries.

Vinegar dissolved a Stone of 3 gr into a Jelly in 10 days in a cold digestion and a 3 gr. fragment in 3 days in a warm digestion. Mountain wine and Red Port did not dissolve the Stone wn. digested 3 days and upwards with it warm.

Honey & water acted upon it a little.

New River water not at all after 3 days digestion 11 hours of which was warm.

Chapt. Vii

Exp. 38 A 4½ gr. calculus being digested in 2 oz of Asparagus Roots for 23 days, easily separated into powder. Juce of Parsley leaves had some effect upon the stones and little or more upon others.

The Apple called Golden Rennet has very little of a quality dissolvent of ye Stone either ye Juce or Decoction.

The decoction of Golden Pippins is in some measure lithotroptick. Also ye Nonparell, but more the Decoction than juce.

Chapt. Viii

Bread has an excellent Lithotriptick Quality as appears from Stones digested in the Infusion of it. I am acquainted with two Gent. who eat some dry Bread in a morning as a Remedy against the Stone.

Small London Beer did not act upon Calculi: nor Porter, in a warm digestion for 3 days.

Infs. of Green Tea did not exert any Lithotriptick quality in 7 days digestion, 27 hours of which was warm. Neither does it appear from his Exp. that Coffee diserves a place amongst the Dissolvents. Altho tis said by Ray, Hist.—Plant: & D. Dufour on Coffee, & Muis & others that some have found great relief in Nephritick Ailments from the use of Coffee. Chocolate & Cocoa have Lithotriptick quality.

Exp. LXIV A 1¾ gr calculus was digested warm 2 days in 2 oz Milk; the Stone was dissolved but the Milk coagulated as thick as Custard.

Exp. LXV A calculus weighing 1 gr. was digested 6 days & 30 hours of it warm in 2 oz of milk & became so soft that it easily rubd into Sand.

Lobb. Chapt. IX

Juce & Decoction of Cabbage especially red seems in some small degree Lithotriptick rendering Stones somewhat softer, this virtue more in the Decoction, than Juce.

Carrots act on Calculi much as Cabbage.

Cellery is a pretty active dissolvent.

Cucumbers have a quality strongly dissolvent, their Juce breaking the Stone into coarse Sand once in 3 days, once in 6 days.

Juce of red Currants, red Currant Wine & ye same Wine mixt with New River Water, did not act upon Calculi.

A Calculus 4½ gr. digested with 2 oz of a decoction of foreign currants 3 days 28 hours of it warm became soft & easily divided into pieces wch rub'd into fine Sand.

He tried many Experiments upon Calculi, with the Juce & Decoctions etc. of various other Vegetable Substances the Events of wch Exp: he hath very accurately related. He at last divides the Substances wherewith he made the Exp. into three general Classes, of wch follows an Abstract.

N.B: J. signifies Juces & D. Decoction.

CLASS I. Containing the stronger dissolvents of the Stone, viz. whereby the Stone was either wholly dissolved, or at least its texture broken.

Bread its infusion
Cellery J & D
Codlins J
Cucumbers J
Currants, foreign D
*Cyder of various kinds
Figgs D
Grapes White J
Hops D
*Leeks J & D & Infusion
Lettice Cabbage J
Limons J
*Milk
Mulberrries J
Mulberry Wine
Non-Parells D
*Onions
Oranges, Seville & China J
Pears Burgamot J
Punch with Honey
Radishes Garden J
Raisins D
Sorrel Common & Wood J
Turnips J D
Green Tea D but not Infusion
Vinegar
Wine White Port.
D° with water

*=Strongest

CLASS II. Containing Weaker dissolvents of the Stone with some of wch ye Stone was softened, at other times broke or hard or dissolved by the same.

Asparagus Roots J
Cabbage White & Red J & D
Carrots J
Coco D
Coffee
Chocolate
Cyder Glostershire & Southam
Elderberry J
Golden Pippin J & D
Golden Rennet D
Hydromel
Mallow leaves J & D
Malt & Hops D
Mulberry, Brandy & Water
Wormwood, Lemon Juce & mineral water.
Non Perell Tea
Onion
Parsley Roots J, D Inf.
D° leaves D inf.
Parsnips J D
Potatoes J D
Barley pearl D
Rice D
Strawberries J Brandy
Tea Bohea Decoction
D° Green D
Wine Red Port
Wine Tent*
Wine Elderberry & Water
Wine Canary
Wine Madeira
Wine Rhenish
Wine Yeast & Water

[*Wine Tent=Spanish red wine of low alcohol]

CLASS III. Things tried wch discovered no quality dissolvent of the Stone.

Barley
Beer Small
D° Porter
Cabbage red J
Horse Radish Root D
Malt D
Millet seeds D
Olives D
Onion Tea
Parsley Root Tea
Rue J
Salt of Wormwood & Water
Spinach J & D
Tea Green Infusion
Verjuce*
D° with Water
Water New River
Water St. Pauls pump
Wheat D
Wine Currant
Wine Elderberry
Wine Leek
Wine Mountain
Wine Rhenish

[*Verjuce=unripe grapes]

[Latin]

August 6th, 1739

79 Mrs. Harriman, of Workington, suffering from pulmonary congestion. A woman of 43, married but infertile, with a robust body, afflicted for many years with an immoderate flow of monthly blood. In the last two or three years her menstrual flow has been temporarily relieved, but has flowed sparingly.

She suffered from very troublesome coughs for the last two years, which brought up vomit and phlegm. Material was brought up with hawking and coughing, thick, viscous and plentiful, thickest in the morning, and this material also fell copiously from her nose into her throat. Her breathing, however, is adequately produced but sometimes it requires a great effort. She has a slight and thready pulse; tongue scurfy and whitish after sleep; profuse sweats break out; appetite is slight; bowels normal; colour good but she was very thin due to the sickness lasting for a long time.

Spring waters should be among her drinks. Her whole body to be rubbed well morning and evening. She must take frequent exercise and especially exercise herself diligently by riding. Welsh flannel to be worn on her stomach and chest. Clothing to be thick. Her diet to be carefully chosen.

Ammoniac gum 2½ scruples; Gum of myrrh 2½ scruples; Opopanax 1½ scruples; Liquorice extract 2 scruples; Best saffron ½ scruple; Flower of benzoin ½ scruple; Wormwood 12 gr; Aniseed oil 12 drops; Sassafras oil 12 drops; Copaiba balsam.
Mix together accurately, make into a lump and from this make 10 pills of 1 drachm each. Take 2 four times a day at 7 and 11 in the morning, 5 in the afternoon, and when going to bed. Take 4 spoonfuls of the following and diligently continue to use hourly until the whole amount is taken.

Shavings of guaiacum 6 oz; Shavings of red sandalwood 1 oz; Root of flowering iris 1½ oz; root of elecampane 1½ oz; Root of sea holly 1½ oz; Crushed raisins 2 oz; Tartar salts 1 scruple. Boil gently for an hour in a closed vessel in spring water to make up to 4 pts. After boiling add:
White hoarhound leaves 1 scruple; Hyssop 1 scruple; Ground ivy 1 scruple; Shavings of sassafras wood 1½ oz; Liquorice root 1½ oz. Make a cold apozem, strain and add: Strong cinnamon water 3 oz. Place the apozem in a cold place and use.
Boil these ingredients in spring water to make up 4 pts and drink this second apozem for her ordinary posset with sweet honey.

80 Mr. Robert Gale, aged about 19, a young man of good character and serious nature, dedicated to the study of books. Born of a father who struggled against the misery of a disease of the hypochondrium which came to a crisis that was resolved by diarrhoea. The young man himself was so affected by rickets in childhood that by the age of 5 he was unable to walk. This weakness persisted from that time and his body was also feeble. At 16 he travelled to Virginia but suffered all during his journey from diarrhoea and when he returned home, he was prostrated by a combination of wasting and weakness. He was also tormented by profuse sweatings day and night. Boerhaave was consulted on this affliction, with the following advice [the following, written in English, is a translation of Boerhaave's consultation]:

I have well considered the description of the case concerning the disposition of these young bodies to profuse sweating. This symptom is caused by a weakness of the vessels and a dissolution of the humours. To correct it I think necessary:

1. To rub al the body with dry hot flannels every morning after sleeping, half an hour.
2. To take care that the bed, the linnen, the Clouds all wel dry.
3. Good deal of Exercise will do much good evicting only the sweating.
4. It shall be very propre to take every three hours of the day three pills A. with a spoonfull of the Liquor B. All these six weeks.

Leyden 17 $\frac{4}{10}$ 37 H. Boerhaave.

A. Catechu 1 drachm; Mastich 1 drachm; Olibanum 1 drachm; Powdered refined sugar 1 drachm; Turpentine 9 drops. Make pills of 3 gr.

B. Distilled salvia water 2 pts; Spirits of wild chamomile 4 oz; Grated salvia 2 oz. Heat until almost boiling in a tall chemical flask for 24 hours, then strain the liquid remaining.

[Brownrigg's own following up of the case continues.]

With the use of these remedies he grew a little better. Next summer he went to Holland but he suffered the whole voyage from diarrhoea again and his strength was noticeably reduced. Last winter, however, he suffered from the nervous fever already described, which greatly increased the weakness. He stayed in the country almost all summer, regularly exercising on horseback. He was still troubled with these profuse sweatings. I also noticed a small dry cough which became frequent with rapid convulsive movements affecting his limbs and lower jaw and he became very weak and depressed in spirit.

Elixir of myns: vitriol 1 oz; Grains of pepper 20.
Take at 11 a.m., 4 p.m. and at bedtime with 5 spoonfuls of the following:
Powdered Peruvian bark 2 oz; Elecampane root 3 scruples; Cochineal 15 gr; Wormwood 2 scruples. Boil for 1 hour in spring water. Make up 2 pts; at the end of the boiling add:
Leaves of St. John's wort 2 pecks; Orange peel 2 scruples; Sassafras 1½ scruples; Root of wild valerian 6 scruples; Root of sagapenum 1 scruple. Strain and add:
Tincture of Dutch grape wine 2 oz; Strong cinnamon water 2 oz. Make the apozem and take as ordered.

3 September, 1739.

81 Mr. David Harris, jaundiced. A robust sailor about 26, in good bodily condition. Affected with jaundice after intermittent fever. I cured him with the following remedies.

> Electuary of rhubarb 2 scruples; Saffron 2 scruples; Vitriolated tartar 1½ scruples; Calcined eggshell ½ oz; Powdered millipede; Electuary of myrrh ½ oz; Conserve of Roman wormwood 1½ oz; Pink syrup.
>
> Root of turmeric; Tincture of madder; Sea holly; Bark of red sandalwood. Boil for ¼ hour, then add:
> Venetian soap 2 oz. Boil, then strain and to 2 pts add: Strong cinnamon water 3 oz; Spirit of lavender 3 oz. Take 1½ spoonfuls.

[This addition is written in English, upside down, at the foot of the page:]

John Hawkins at the Sign of the Dragoon in the Roperie. Jane Marr.

[This case is written in English.]

82 Mrs. Waters,[169] dropsy of the chest, rheumatism, cachexia, etc.

To Dr. Salkeld.

Mrs. Waters, a Gentlewoman aged about 49, of a full habit of Body, having born six or seven children, for many years past very infirm, seldom enjoying a tolerable State of Health, having been much afflicted with the Rhumatism, Gravel, Asthma, Dropsical swellings in her Leggs and several other Disorders for which she had taken a great variety of Remedies.

About the latter end of May last when I first saw her she complained of flying rhumatick Pains, and pains in the Head a continual pain and weight at her Stomach, and a very great difficulty in breathing which was much increased by motion, she breathed short but without any great noise or motion of the breast, and did not seem to be much troubled with a Cough or Phlegm, her Leggs were also a little swelled.

For these complaints I ordered some Pills with the Gum and Soap; and apozem with the wood and roots of elecampane-spirit; Liquorice etc as also a mixture with Oxymel of Squills.

These being constantly taken for some time did not seem to give her any relief. I therefore advised constant Riding in the Country Air, with a proper diet. She constantly found herself much refreshed by riding but the complaints still continued.

Towards the latter end of June she told me that upon mounting on Horseback she had for some time perceived her heart to heave as if it were loose in her breast, and that it gave her great uneasiness but settled after riding, this gave me some suspicion of a hydrops pectoris. A more strict inquiry being therefore made, I was confirmed in my opinion so as not to doubt that this was the occasion of the Asthma. For she not only perceived this fluctuation in her Breast upon riding or any other quick motion, but also when she stooped forward. The load and continual pain which she said she felt at her stomach, extended quite round

[169] Mary, wife of William Waters who provided the fir used to make pipes for the pumps for the Newcomen engine at Saltom Pit. She died 21st December 1739, aged 48.

from the Scrobiculus Cordis to the Back, she describing to be seated exactly in the parts where the Diaphragm is connected to the Ribs, and therefore seemed to be occasioned by the weight and pressure of the Water upon the Diaphragm. The Asthma was also least in the Evenings, and after she went to bed gradually increased so that she seldom slept unless it was immediately after she gott into bed, and was often constrained to sit up in the nights and had constantly a great Struggle for Breath in the Morning. The Manner of breathing being short and without any great Noise or motion of the Breast, seemed to show that the difficulty proceeded from a Compression of the Lungs.

Thinking that this watery Humour might probably be expelled by diureticks I therefor prescribed a Venereal Tincture made in Sal Volatile and Olive Oil: which I had experienced to be a powerfull diuretick deobstruent and which I gave at first in small quantities gradually increasing the dose. This promoted a plentifull discharge by Urine by which she seemed to be much releived.

But about the beginning of July catching cold she was siezed with a fever and a violent pain in her side, accompanied with an incessant cough, which complaints yielded to Aperient decoctions, Nitrous Remedies, cooling Purges and Fomentations. For some time after she continued resolved to make no further use of Remedies, but afterwards was desirous of having recourse to them again being wearied with her disorder which had increased so much that she breathed with the greatest difficulty.

On Aug. 6th at her desire a Blister was therefore applyed which she said had formerly releived her when she was held in much the same way.

I also ordered her some diuretick Ingredients of the Alcaline kind such as Root of Radish; Millepede; beans; Salt; Wormwood infused in Wine with Gentian and other Stomaticks. Observing that she grew very thirsty and that her Tongue was very dry and black and that she complained of a great heat and uneasiness after she took this remedy I therefore desired her to make no further use of it. Being importuned to prescribe further I ordered her a strong purge with Root of black bindweed: wch had a much better effect than I expected. I therefore repeated it six or eight times by which means she was enabled to breath with a great ease and freedom the last purge she took about the 10 of 7^{br}. I then again tryed Corroborants but found that they would not agree with her since they increased the Heat and Thirst Dryness and blackness of the Tongue still remaining. Since that time I have only advised Spirit of Nitre or Nitrous powders, she also takes a large Dose of Laudanum every night wch makes her life tolerably easy *altho I have offtimes diswaded the use of it.*[170] Since she left of the use of her Purges her Leggs and all the lower parts are swelled with water to a most enormous bulk, her Belly is also much distended, she breathes with a little more ease than formerly, but says that she finds a great Vacuity or emptiness about her Breast which is very troublesome to her. The discharge by Urine is greater than could be expected under these Circumstances, all the other natural discharges have also been regular, except perhaps that of Persperation. Her pulse now is and all ways has been very good. She has had a tolerable good Stomach till of late, *but tis now very bad.*[171]

[170] The words between the asterisks were inserted later.

[171] The words between the asterisks were inserted later.

These are the most material Circumstances, altho she is troubled with the Haemorrhoids, Lumbago Rheumatica and many other complaints too hidous to mention.
W.B.

10. 8^{bris} 1739.

Dr. Salkeld seemed to commend what had been done and advised her to continue the use of the purges, taken every other day, using Nitrous powders on the intermediate days, and entirely dissaproved the use of Laudanum; she took several purges but to no purpose, as they only weakened her, so that at length she was obliged to desist; and died about the 21st of December having been affected with a Delirium and Coma for about a week before her death.[172]

October 18th, 1739

83 Mrs. William Gale, a gentlewoman, blessed with many virtues, about 36 or 38 when she married, of good bodily constitution, but plump and obese. In the first years of her marriage she always miscarried about the third month of her pregnancy. At about forty, she bore first a daughter, then a son, then a daughter. By last April, after a break of 7 years, she conceived again, or so she supposed. Her suspicions of conception arose due to the following phenomena. Her age was now over 50 and her periods which had always flowed regularly, suddenly stopped. Before this change she had observed no other external cause, other than that she was cast down by the death of her mother and had been confined to bed with this great grief. Now, with the failure of her periods, she was attended with morning sickness and all the symptoms of being pregnant. After the 18th September, the break in her periods ceased and she had a constant flow for 3 or 4 days. To stop the flow, I carried out a venesection and gave her other remedies to stop it. At the end of the next month the flow has now returned again, but she is in no doubt that she is still pregnant as her lower abdomen was occupied by a growth just like a foetus, and she felt it moving like a child at the normal time. I prescribed restringents to use for this and after 3 or 4 days the flow stopped.[173]

[These prescriptions for Mrs. Gale were later written on small sheets and pasted in the Casebook.]

Toasted rhubarb root 6 gr; Powdered amber 6 gr; Catechu 5 gr; Powdered bloodstone ½ scruple; Cinnamon oil.

Powdered bloodstone, Peruvian bark, finely powdered; Powdered amber; Toasted rhubarb; Confection of Fracastoro; Conserve of red rose; Balsamic syrup. Make an electuary the size of a nutmeg. Take first thing in the morning and when going to bed. Take 2 spoonfuls of the julep above. 2 other spoonfuls if required.

10th May 1740.
Gum ammoniac 2½ scruples; Myrrh 2½ scruples; Opopanax 1 scruple; Best saffron 2 scruples; Borax 2 scruples; Pill ruffi 1 scruple; Extract of gentian 4 scruples; Juniper oil 25 drops.

[172] This paragraph is a later insertion.

[173] A woman at the menopause with menstrual irregularity who decided she was pregnant, but bleeding restarted after six months. As in some other cases Brownrigg does not tell us the end of the story.

This quantity of elixir will be made into pills of 5 gr. Three of these should be taken at 10 a.m., 5 p.m., and when going to bed.
5 spoonfuls of the following apozem:
Root of fresh burberry 3 oz; China root 3 scruples; Sarsaparilla 3 scruples; Bark of red sandalwood shaved 3 scruples; Vitriolated tartar 2 scruples;
Boil for half an hour in pure water. Make up 2 pts. Add after final straining:
Dandelion root 2½ oz; Root of sea holly 3 scruples; Juniper berries 1½ oz.
Strain and forcibly squeeze, and to the remaining deposit add:
Strong cinnamon water 1½ oz; Gum ammoniac; Myrrh; Opopanax; Saffron; Borax; Extract of gentian; Juniper oil; Pill Ruffi; Strasbourg turpentine; Proprietory elixir.

Fresh burdock root; Dandelion; China; Sarsaparilla; Sandalwood; Vitriolated tartar.
Boil for ½ an hour in spring water. Make up 2 pts and add after straining:
Juniper berries 1½ oz; Liquorice root 6 scruples; Sea holly; Sassafras wood shavings 6 scruples. Strain and add Strong cinnamon water 3 oz.

[This page is full of fragments written in English at different times, mainly on some scientific observations. These may be concerned with his early work on the fire damp with Carlisle Spedding.]

a) Resistance in Air itself therefore not perfectly fluid. A small Cohesion or none at all it is necessary that they should not touch at all or only by a few points. Exp. Vacuities necessary. Particles of most fluid have Agitation Those [illegible] wch repell. Are not live therefore absolutely necessary tho to keep the parts of Bodies separate, to d., into minute parts and to agitate them and

b) There
The requisites to Fluidity are first minuteness of Parts

——

Thus Exemp:

c) Observation holds goods of all liquids [upside down]

d) Bodies may have a propre figure and a very Cohesion, and yet wanting a smallness of parts form a fluid (for while they retain a sensible [illegible]) because great Particles will require a considerable force to fuel them and a still greater force is necessary to set parts out of their way, hard and resisting. Conditions very opposite. But their Condition alone is not sufficient particle of Smoke is much grosser than a part being may be resolved compounded of Earth, Oil, Salt and waters.

——

Corpuscles how formed-
How rendered more unfit. Exemp: in the whole of A third requisite for Fluidity.
Many things inexplicable. Ex. in Ob. F. & W.

e) [written upside down]
gather, We also may learn the great (absolute) necessity fire or Heat to enter into the composition (needing subtile rarifies) to open in promoting fluidity is so great.
They act as solvent not only by destroying the Cohesion
-very mina
of fluidity owing

f) Sea holly, Squills, Tartar, Aniseed [written over at right angles later on].

84 To Miss Cookson of Newcastle.

A girl of 20, her mother and all her family were prone to melancholy. She herself for several years suffered irregular periods with little flow. Now her periods had entirely stopped for 5 months. She was afflicted with melancholy and almost perpetual insomnia.

[Below is a copy of a letter in English which Brownrigg sent to her.]

Madam, Whitehaven 9 March 1739/40.

I am sorry by your sudden departure I was deprived of the opportunity of seeing you before you left Whitehaven, having found that you were unexpectedly gone when I called in the morning to take my leave. I here return my thanks for your favour and have sent my Sentiments of your disorder, with directions for such Remedies as I think most proper in your Case. These I submit for Consideration of some prudent Physician who can have frequent Opportunities of visiting you, and can Vary his prescriptions as accidental Circumstances may require. I think your Case absolutely requires that you should put yourself under the Care of some such Gentleman as I have described, the approaching Season of the year encouraging me to expect that all your Complaints may then by proper methods be removed, but should this opportunity be neglected a cure could not be attempted at another Season with equal hopes of success. I sincerely wish you a perfect Recovery of your Health and am

Madam,

Your most Obedient Servant,

W. B.

[Below is a copy, written in Latin, of his case observations. This would have been enclosed with Miss Cookson's letter.]

Miss Cookson is affected by a long standing suppression of her periods which has resulted in a weakness in her organs of digestion and concoction. The blood is crude and not properly produced, poorly adapted to circulating or the necessary secretions: her animal spirits are wrongly produced; blood deposited in the liver where they stagnate; from there originate the blockage and obstruction of the viscera. That this is so is clearly shown by the trembling and shaking limbs, spontaneous insomnia, pale skin, whitish stools, weariness, emotional upsets and other phenomena.

Thus the most fitting remedies for these symptoms would seem to be those to remove the thick and stagnant humours and make them more ready for movement, to open the full and obstructed viscera and at the same time strengthen the solid structures in the body. For food, she should take easily digestible things and water fairly mixed with white wine for her everyday drink. For other drinks she should carefully abstain from tea and coffee in the afternoon. Regular riding on an empty stomach will exercise the body and by this exercise sleep will be encouraged, rather than by the use of narcotics, which in this case I in no way recommend. Rubbing all the abdomen with woollen cloth morning and night will be of great value.

The following, or similar, should be administered:

Pure native gum ammoniac 2 scruples; Gum galbanum 2 scruples; Gum of myrrh 2 scruples; Venetian soap 1½ scruples; Electuary of rhubarb 1 scruple; Saffron ½ scruple;

Gentian extract 2 scruples; Amber oil 18 drops; Savin oil 18 drops; Strasbourg turpentine. Make up a mass for the pills and make each one 1 drachm. Make 12 pills and take 3 a day at 11 a.m., 5 p.m. and at bedtime. These to be followed by 2 spoonfuls of wine mixture: Root of angelica 3 scruples; Root of hyssop 3 scruples; Root of gentian 3 scruples; Zedoar 1½ scruples; Extract of orange 1½ scruples; Sassafras bark 2 scruples; Wormwood 3½ scruples; Cochineal 1 scruple; Old vintage Rhenish wine up to 2 pts. Stand warm for 48 hrs in a well-sealed flask. Strain the wine and use as directed above.

The patient should persist in this method until it becomes clear from signs known to the wise physician that the free movement of the viscera of the abdomen has been achieved. There can also be correctly applied more strengthening remedies which strongly promote menstruation, especially chalybeated Rhenish wine, Ens Veneris and similar aperient ferrous preparations.

Redundant humours should be channelled back to the lower areas and the contracting uterine vessels can be relaxed in a similar manner by the use of footbaths, inhalants and rubbing.

If these remedies do not stop this illness then about the beginning of June, ferrous mineral waters (those from Tunbridge Wells and numerous others of a similar type which are located almost everywhere) must be brought back into use. For these healthgiving waters, drunk at the spring under the guidance of a good doctor, promoting a normal evacuation, are extremely good at opening the blocked viscera and at strengthening the whole body.

I humbly submit all these to the judgment of more experienced doctors.

Whitehaven. 8 March 1739/40 W. Brownrigg.

OF THE CONESSI BARK[174]

[English section.]

The Cort. Conessi, or Conessi-seca is the bark of a tree not unlike the Cadogapala of the Malabars. It is brought from the East Indies, and is an excellent Remedy in Dysenteries: general evacuations being first made as bleeding, Vomiting with Ipecacuanha; or purging with Rhubarb according to the nature of the Case. Of this Bark, half a drachm finely powdered made into a bolus with orange syrup is to be taken four times a day. The first day it usually increases the number of stools, but without increasing the Gripings, and will generally cure obstinate Dysenteries in 4 or five days time. It also cures such as are troubled with an habitual diarrhoea in moist rainy weather.

The Electuary must be made fresh every day, or every other day, because it soon loses its taste and Virtue. After the Dysentery is stopped, the patient will sometimes be affected with violent pains between the Shoulders & which are best removed by bleeding.

Mr. Monroe had this acc[t] from a Gent: who had been a long time in the E. Indies, and confirms it partly by his own Experience, having with it quickly cured an obstinate and inveterate Diarrhoea.

See *Medical Essays*. Vol. 3, page 32.[175]

[174] The bark of Wrightia antidysenterica (Conessi Cortex).

[175] A. Monro, 'An account of the effects of the Conessi Bark', *Medical Essays and Observations*, Edinburgh, 1735, vol. 3, pp. 32–5.

[Latin section. Brownrigg has put an insertion in the margin to indicate that this should really follow the French section.]

Such true dysentery is horrible and this sickness is very common in these regions, killing more of the people than another unnatural affection. If, when the symptoms are severe, the pain excruciating and in the long time of the crisis the patient is not to die, one should have recourse to extract of Saffron, than which, I dare to say, no more suitable remedy can be devised by human thought. I regard this as the true antidote to this illness feared though it may often be.

Bontius. *On the Medicine of the Indies*, page 23, 24.[176]

[French section.]

Dysenteries of all kinds are common, difficult, dangerous and even result in death, not only in the Indies but also on voyages. I was displeased to see that the remedies I used produced little effect and I desired to discover anything which would alleviate the suffering of my patients. At last I had the good fortune to meet someone who had lived in the Indies for several years, who had used a remedy which was easy to prepare and take. With the use and correct treatment of this, I have cured a very great number of people in the Indies, on voyages and in France since my return. To see that an invalid is not reduced to the final extremity, even though he is ill, must cheer him a little.

Dr. Dillon [*sic*]. *Voyage to the East Indies.* Chapter on dysenteries, page 303.[177]

[Brownrigg's observation in Latin:]

Does not this remedy seem to be the Conessi Bark?

[English section.]

Mr. John Gale of W^{t}haven sent a parcel of the Conessi Bark from the East Indies to his father Mr. Elisha Gale, he gave it extraordinary eulogies for its great Vertues in curing Fluxes of all kinds, wch he said it infallibly removed after bleeding; he also said it cured agues, and desired that his brother Joseph might never go to sea without it. As the Gent: who sent this acc^{t} was not very inquisitive, it thence appears that the Conessi Bark is a remedy commonly known in the E. Indies, and is much used, and highly estemeed for curing those violent Dysenteries wherewith they are so often afflicted there.

It is a bark in appearances not much unlike the Peruvian Bark but of a darker colour. Its taste doth also resemble that of the Peruvian Bark, but it is a far stronger, Bitter, more pungent and less rough upon the tongue. It seems to possess an anodine quality because it is observed to ease the pains. Besides its restringent and corroborating virtues, it is also moderately detergent as appears from its increasing the number of stools on the first day.

[176] Jacopus Bontius, *De medicina Indorum*, in P. Alpinus, *De medicina Aegyptiorum*, Paris, N. Redelichuysen, 1645.

[177] C. Dellon, *Nouvelle relation d'un voyage fait aux Indes orientales*, Amsterdam, F. Marret, 1699.

85 Miss Kitty Griffiths, persistent dysentery cured by the Conessi Bark. A young woman of about 28, and according to nature, of a good and robust constitution of body. In the spring of 1739 she was seized by a violent dysentery in Edinburgh and evacuated a large amount of blood mixed with stools. In that place, use was made of various remedies first, then restringents. She travelled to Cumberland and there took several remedies prescribed by Dr. Carlyle and she went horse riding for exercise. With these she was given some occasional relief from her complaint, but she was not completely cured. It recurs if the slightest mistake is made in the six non-naturals, and is particularly oppressive in the morning after a tormented night.I noted her stools were broken up by the onset of the illness and were no longer bloody, but watery. In this way, the condition was prolonged to the beginning of January 1739/40, by which time I was called, noting the patient's considerable weakness and wasting and that her illness was rejecting the remedies. I therefore prescribed the following, by which she was relieved immediately from the stomach cramps and the diarrhoea was swiftly checked. The illness was entirely cured by repeating the course of medicines once only.

Root of ipecacuanha powdered ½ scruple; Rue water 1½ oz; Syrup of violet 1 scruple. Make a draught. Take at 4 p.m. with each regime.
Conessi bark powdered finely ½ oz, Nutmeg 2 scruples; Andromachus treacle 1½ scruples; Marmalade for flavour. Make the electuary. Take the amount of a nutmeg 3 times daily at noon, followed by 5 spoonfuls of:
Red sandalwood 2 oz; Sarsaparilla root 5 scruples; Salt of tartar ½ scruple. Boil for quarter of an hour in spring water then add:
Husks of juniper berries 2½ oz; Shavings of sassafras wood 1½ oz. Boil in a closed flask; strain 2 pts and add: Strong cinnamon water 2 oz.

[Written in English.]

86 Mrs. Christian, Unerigg.[178] Persistent Diarrhoea.
Her own Account of her Case as sent to Dr. Mead.

S^r^

I am 42 years old, mother of 5 Children at 26 till which time I had very good Health, but after that I often miscarried, tho' never after I was 10 weeks gone; that brought the Hysterick Illness upon me, which affected me with lowness of Spirits, a bad appetite and sometimes a violent pain in the right side, or else the Toothake. I slept very little which brought me to the use of Laudanum but tho' I have used it 15 years I seldom take more than 20 or 25 drops, While I was so apt to miscarry, I was subject to flood, and lost too much at other certain times but for 10 years past I have not exceeded that way. Upon taking proper Remedies I always recovered, and then fell with Child, and if I recovered well perhaps had another Child before I relapsed. Ten years ago I had the Measels, which I hardly recovered. That quite altered my very nature, for before that I was always costive, but since that have been very subject to a looseness, which is my greatest trouble at present. Tho I have had four children since, three of which are living and healthfull, I was

[178] She was Bridget Senhouse of Netherhall, Maryport, who married John Christian of Unerigg (or Ewanrigg). He was the 14th head of the Christian family of Milntown, Isle of Man, and a barrister by profession. They had 11 living children, one of whom, Charles, was the father of the *Bounty* mutineer, Fletcher Christian.

always the worst when I was with Child, and very much troubled with Looseness the first week after I was delivered, but after that allways recovered very well. I have taken many Remedies which helped me a little, but as soon as I was better, I fell with Child and then was the same thing as before. I drank Tea made with the Woods a long time, but could not find any alteration from it. It is near two years since I bore my last Child, and my appetite has never been so good as it was before, and my Looseness and other Ailments have been worse. I am allways the worst from May to November, and am the best in the Spring. Very often the day before I am loose, I am very much loaden and dull, then perhaps I have five or six Stools, but not allways very loose, but it is more than I can bear as I eat little; then I take Laudanum and am fine after it; the next day I seldom go to Stool, the third day, perhaps, I go twice, and the 4th day I am loose again and take Laudanum; but this is when I am the very best; but sometimes it returns every day, but that is not often; sometimes in Summer it is attended with Colick pains, but not often. For 7 years last I have had my natural disorder once in three weeks which continues 6 or 7 days. Before and after and in the middle of that time I am more than commonly loose besides I am a little troubled with the whites, both before and after that disorder; so that I am never many days free from one of those troubles. Notwithstanding, I have been slenderer, apter to take cold, and weaker than I am at present. Tho I am naturally chearfull and have very good Spirits, and when I am well of an easy temper, yet when I am ill, my Spirits are greatly affected, and cannot help fretting at everything; especially in a morning. I am always better towards night, and sleep tolerably well w^{h} I am no way disturbed; but Grief or Joy or Weariness takes my sleep away. I have taken Vitriol Drops of late, I cannot say it helped my Appetite much, but I was easier after eating since I took it; tho I found no other Alteration, except it was the Case that the last time, I was a week longer betwixt my natural disorder than usual, and all that week I was loose; but now am the same as I commonly have been. For the last year I have taken a Drachm of toasted Rhubarb once in a month or five weeks; I am always better and lightsomer after it; but it makes no Alteration as to the looseness. I was so grievously troubled with the Tooth-ake for many years, that at last I chewed Tobacco, wch I have done for seven years and more. My teeth are very much decayed but never ake since, but are a little sore sometimes, and my face will swell a bit sometimes but without pain; but has been better since I took Rhubarb. I live regular and eat but little beef or mutton; Veal, Fouls or Broath or pudding, Eggs or Roots, etc. are my Diet. Tea has mostly been my breakfast, but not strong. For some years I have drank water in Summer and often a Glass of Wine after it, and Beer or small Ale in Winter but I am never thirsty.

I take my illness to be Hysterick and a bad habit of Body, and I think if any thing could help my Stomach and bring me to be regular in going to Stool, every other Complaint would vanish in course.

The reason of this bad habit I take to be falling with Child in ten days time after the Measels went of, I miscarried when that Child was but 15 weeks old, and was delivered of another Child 41 weeks after I miscarried, so that I was three times with Child and had had the Measels in less than a year and an half, and being often loose, and taking Laudanum to stop it without other Remedies, has fixed it.

Dr. Mead's answer to the foregoing Case directed to Mr. Clementson.

Ormond Street, Nov[r] 6, 1739.

S[r]

I have your Account of the Case of a Gentlewoman of 42 with a Diarrhoea etc., I have carefully considered it, and as the whole habit of body seems to be concerned in this Indisposition, I think that must be mended before this Discharge from the Intestines can be brought into right order, I would therefore advise the following method, which should be continued for two or three months:

> Root of Ipecacue 1 scruple; Milky Alexandrine water 1½ oz; Clove of pink syrup 1 scruple.
> Make the draught: take it in the morning with orange juice very weak between vomiting.
>
> Conserve of red roses 1½ oz; Red coral crushed 2 scruples; Diamber specific 1 scruple; Crocus martis well levigated 1½ scruples; with syrup and skin of Orange. Make the electuary. Take a quantity the size of a large nutmeg in the morning and at 5 in the afternoon. Bristol water warmed ½pt.
>
> Mixed herbs 2 scruples; Coral (red) powdered & toasted nutmeg (each ½ scruple); Toasted rhubarb 6 gr; Liquid Laudanum 8 drops; Crocus syrup. Make up Pills, take every night when retiring 4 spoonfuls of red wine. Repeat the emetic draught once a week.

She must forbear all Malt Liquors, and make her common Drink, Bristol Water with a little red Wine.

I am S[r] yo[r] most Humble Serv[t].

Dr. Mead.

She took the Remedies above prescribed by Doct[r] Mead untill the beginning of April 1740. But not percieving any benefit from then I was called on Ap. the 1st. She told me that the Vomits seemed to disagree with her exceedingly, and allways left a great weakness and lowness of Spirits and want of Appetite, that the other Remedies were not unpleasant but sometimes seemed to bind her too much, and then she w[d] have a swelling in her face, and flying Pains untill the Diarrhoea returned, which it frequently did as before, notwithstanding the Use of the Restringent Remedies. That in other respects she had been much the same as formerly. That she once took by Dr Senhouse's Directions an Infusion of Peruvian Bark; and other Ingredients in Wine w[ch] she thought was the most serviceable of anything she has taken.

Several facts observed by me

She is of the Senhouses of Netherhall, a strong, healthy and long lived Family; her Children are also healthy; she is tall, and has a fair clear complexion; she is rather lean than otherwise, but is no way emaciated. She never had any Leucophlegmatick Swellings; but is of an exceedingly soft, lax and spongy Habit of body and consequently perspires little. Of a lively Disposition, but of so delicate a frame that she is much affected by the lightest Cause; so that she can bear no cold or any other alteration, therefore almost constantly confines herself at home, and can seldom ride out without finding some disorder after it. There is no fault in her Pulse or Respiration.

[Brownrigg's later note:]

I ordered the following Remedies:

[Small page inserted.]

For Mrs. Christian.

Powdered crabs eyes 1½ scruples; Powdered red coral 1½ scruples; White powdered amber 1½ scruples; Finely powdered Peruvian bark 2 scruples; Astringent crocus martis 2 scruples; Well beaten ginger root 6 scruples; Conserve of golden orange 1 oz; syrup and skin of orange. Make an electuary and take an amount the size of a nutmeg before breakfast, at 11 a.m. and at dinner. Take daily. Take 3 & 4 spoonfuls of this following infusion like tea:
Galingale root 1 scruple; Zedoar root 1 scruple; Cinnamon bark 2 scruples; Dried orange skin 2 scruples; Red sandalwood bark shavings ½ oz; Lemon ½ oz; Sassafras ½ oz; Juniper berries. Cut up, grind and divide the mixture and pour equally into 6 papers. Take 1 paper in 1 pt boiled river water like tea.

[Written on a page of the Casebook.]

Mrs. Christian. 1 April, 1740.

Electuary of rhubarb root 2½ scruples; Clove pink syrup. Make a bolus and take first thing in the morning; continue with the next measure after a period and finish the remainder at bedtime. Take a dose of liquid laudanum and repeat the bolus after an interval of 2 days, then whenever required. Dried Conessi bark finely powdered ½ scruple; Powdered zedoar bark 2 scruples; powdered best saffron 1 scruple; Andromachus treacle 1½ scruples; Marmalade 3 scruples. Rose syrup. Make an electuary and take a dose the size of a nutmeg at 10 a.m. and 5 p.m.
Take 4 spoonfuls of the following:
Shavings of red sandalwood 2 oz; Root of gentian 2 scruples; Root of sarsaparilla 2 scruples; China root 2 scruples; Salt of tartar ½ scruple. Boil for 1½ hours in spring water, then add: Crushed juniper berries 2 oz; Shavings of sassafras wood 1½ oz; root of galingale 1 scruple; Golden orange 1 scruple. Boil in a closed vessel, then remove from the fire and allow to distill in hot water for 4 hours. Strain 28 oz until clear, then add: Strong cinnamon water 2 oz; Tincture of Dutch grape wine 2 oz.

[English]

It was above a fortnight before she could begin the use of these Remedies, in wch time not taking her Restringent Remedies and having got cold she had a very severe fit of her Looseness wch continued for 4 or 5 days, so that she was obliged to take 40 drops of Laudanum several times, which was more than she ever had taken before.

Mrs. Christian.
Memoirs of her Case wch I did not send to Mrs. Christian.

I have prepared the following wine for Mrs. Christian myself. 2nd October 1740.

Electuary of dried Conessi bark roughly ground 6 scruples; Cinnamon 2 scruples; Golden orange 2 scruples; Root of zedoar 1 scruple; Virginian snake root 1 scruple; Small cardamom seeds 1 scruple; Iron filings 1 scruple; Best red French wine 2 pts.
Divide while straining and take 1 spoonful at 11 a.m. and 2 spoonfuls at 3 p.m. and at bedtime.

Letter and directions sent to Mrs. Christian about a year after the former.
6th April, 1741.

Continue to use the electuary with Conessi bark already described and after a single dose take 3 spoonfuls of the following in place of the decoction:
Dried orange 6 scruples; Root of galingale 2 scruples; Angelica root ½ oz; Spec. diamber 2 scruples; Fresh iron filings 2 oz; Red wine from Portugal 4 pts.
Divide into seven flasks soundly stopped, and then strain for use.

N.B. She complained that this did not agree with her stomach.

[A rough draft, with many corrections, of the letter which must have been sent on 6th April.]

Mad.

According to my Promise I have directed to Mr. Clementson to prepare you some Wine to be used along with the electuary which I formerly prescribed, which I hope will not only instead of ye be kept more conveniently than the decoction, but may also prove more Effectual in removing, or at least in promoting a proper digestion of your food, by strengthening the whole Body, especially the Nervous System by its gentle Restringent quality etc. I should be extreamly rejoyced to find that it agrees with you. The good Effect wch I hope from it, and am with the most hearty Prayers for your Welfare I had the pleasure of Mr. Christian's opinions & may probably have yours.

[Pasted into the Casebook.]

7 Oct. 1742.

I herewith send you some wine wch I thought proper to prepare for you myself, if it agrees with you (as I hope it will) I shall send the prescription for it to Mr. Clementson. The Ingredients are such as are of a very strengthening Nature and I hope may assist y^{r} digestion, strengthen y^{r} Nervous System, and moderately restrain those Evacuations wch are too violent, and properly regulate others. These Ingredients are infused in good French Claret wch I think more light than Port, and better fitted to extract the Virtues of y^{r} Ingred. and better suited to y^{r} case you may strain that wine off from ye Ingredients about Saturday Next. four spoonfulls of it will be sufficient.
to be taken in a day with a spoonfull an hour, before Dinner, 2 Spoonfulls about 4 o Clock in the Afternoon, and a Spoonful going to rest. But, you may begin with taking a single spoonfull in the Afternoon and so taking a little more every day, as you find y^{r} Stomach will bear it. until you come to four Spoonfulls. If you think y^{r} strength will bear it it might be very proper to take a moderate dose of Powder of Rhubarb before you begin with the Use of the Wine. My Spouse joins with in our kind respects to you and Mr Christian she was much delighted wth her Journey, got very well home and thinks herself greatly obliged for the Civility you were pleased to show us as does also dear Mad^{m}.

[A series of small extra sheets pasted over the previous prescriptions and all much later addenda.]

W^{t}haven 4 November, 1742.

(a) Mad^{m}

I was favoured with your letter, and have herewith sent the prescription for the Wine to Mr. Clementson, I am very sorry that you have lately had so greate a disorder upon you. I heartily rejoyce with you that you have overcome your late disorder. If you should ever happen to be again under the like Circumstances, I think it w^{d} be as well to refrain at that time from the use of the Wine, because altho it is moderately restringent, yet being a pretty warm remedy it might at such time rather increase your Disorder than abate it but it may be very proper to take it at any time when you (are) have those Discharges in a moderate way, and I have great hopes that it may be 'servisable' to you for the purpose for wch I formerly recommended it. I think that you might receive some advantage from taking about half a pint of Spa Water, or, rather less every day about one hour before Dinner, especially if you could take a little of y^{r} Wine along with it. I w^{d} not advise you to take a larger quantity than half a pint of it in the forenoon at this cold Season of the year, but it may do very well mixt with Red Wine for your common drink at meals. If you are not provided with any I can procure some for you.

I am glad to hear that Mr. Christian is so well. I beg my humble respects to Mr. Christian. I am very glad to hear that he is so well. I remain you^{r} most obliged and most Humble Servt. I sent to enquire when Mr. Fearon was expected in Town for his mothers sake.

wth wch I beg you w^{d} make Miss Biddy acquainted.

(b) Return papers wch I have considered with the greatest attention. Altho it is not expected/required of a Physician to give his Opinion of the Nature of disease and Reasons for what he does, yet sometimes absolutely necessary if he expects a Complyance, and allways satisfactory if he can so explain himself as to be understood and his method of proceeding appears rational. Nor do I think it is revealing my Art to explain so much to everyone who is capable of understanding as from a good accurate description of y^{r} disease. As I am therefore desirous of doing everything wch may contribute any way to y^{r} satisfaction, I hope you will not be thought too troublesome if I endeavour to give you a short view of my Sentiments of the nature of y^{r} Disorder in as intelligible a manner as the nature of the Subject will admit of.

The first observation wch I shall make is that you have an exceeding soft and lax habit of Body: perhaps the extraordinary evacuations to wch you have been subjected may be the Cause of this Laxity and debility of y^{r} Fibres, but from what ever Cause it proceeds, the Consequence of it will necessarily be That in such a Constitution the Evacuation by perspiration must be exceeding small and much less than it ought. This might be demonstrated by reasoning but will appear more plain to you from facts thus: Children are of a more lax habit of Body than those who are grown up and altho they are not so from so strong a laxture of fibres, perspire less in proportion to the quantity of their food, surplus being expended in their growth. Thus Women who have more soft and lax and weak fibres than Men, and therefore have not so free perspiration the surplus being either expended upon the nourishment of the Foetus, or else discharged at certain regular periods. Men also of a more lax habit of Body have their periodical evacuations either by Vomit, Stool and as I have found by frequent observations, by the fair Sex at a certain time better towards night.

I have attentively considered y^r^ case of wch I think I have a perfect idea from y^r^ Description, I imagine that y^r^ disorder partly proceeds from a too great Laxity and weakness of the Intestines and Viscera Chylopoietica partly from a debility of y^r^ whole Habit of Body, by wch means certain humours are retained wch ought to be carried off by other Evacuations. This is obvious from Heaviness/Lowness of Sp., preceeding the disorder, from the Consequences of the disorder wch During so long a time have not weakened you more.

To strengthen then the whole habit of Body.

To Corroborate and Bind the Intestines.

To Determine the Humours to be evacuated by other natural Evacuations.

(c) Mr. Clementson

Dear Sir:

I here send a prescription for some Wine which Mrs. Christian desires you prepare for her. I beg that you w^d^ endeavour to procure some right good French Claret to prepare it with wch it will be much preferable to Port. Having some good Claret by me I prepared Mrs. Christian a little of it myself for a Trial so that she knows how to take it.

I am y^r^ most Obed^t^ Servant

please to forward the inclosed.

(d) Root of wild valerian 6 scruples; Root of zedoar 1½ scruples; Root of galingale 1½ scruples; Electuary of Peruvian bark roughly powdered ½ scruple. Cinnamon 2½ scruples; Dried orange peel 1½ scruples. Small cardamom seeds 1½ scruples; Iron filings fresh 3 scruples; Rhenish wine 3 pts.

Let them stew together for 3 days, then strain the wine for use. Take 1 spoonful 4 times a day, 1 hour after breakfast, the hour before lunch, 3 p.m. and an hour before dinner.

W. B.

29th September 1743.

[Written in his "best handwriting" to make the instructions clear. Later addition to the bottom:]

She took this often and I thought she received benefit from it, but could only use it in the afternoons because it heated her and disordered her soon after she took it, therefore I directed her as on the other side, [reverse of sheet]

Mrs. Christian

Dried Conessi bark, powdered fine ½ oz; Powdered zedoar 2 scruples; Best saffron 1 scruple; Andromachus treacle 1½ scruples; Marmalade 3 scruples; Syrup of dried roses. Take one piece the size of a nutmeg at 10 a.m. & 5 p.m. and 4 spoonfuls of the following: Red sandalwood shavings 2 oz; Gentian root 2 scruples; Sarsaparilla root 2 scruples; China root 2 scruples; Salt of tartar ½ scruple. Boil for quarter of an hour in spring water then add:
Juniper berries 2 oz; Shavings of sassafras wood 1½ oz; Galingale root 1 scruple; Orange 1 scruple. Boil again.

[Latin]

(e) Mrs. Christian, now aged 49.

Her periods have ceased since last autumn, i.e. September. Until Christmas she was faint and tired every night and gripped with colic pains. In spring and all winter, rheumatic pains for which he cut her vein 3 times, and in spring did this also once, six weeks ago, and she took a rhubarb purgative 3 times with the result that her spirits were depressed for a week. Now when she goes to bed her breathing is comfortable. She sleeps quietly until 2 or 3 in the morning. She feels intense heaviness of her limbs and she has diarrhoea, but without colic pains. She has 3 or 4 evacuations then sweating, and at 6 a.m. the heaviness departs.

[Written at 90 degrees to the above in Latin:]

(f) When her depressed spirit rises she sneezes, coughs, shivers, shakes, expels phlegm and has palpitations and wind, especially through her mild terror, and she takes opium which eases her—in the morning her spirits are good—after lunch internal heaviness—before the diarrhoea there was once colicky pains—leucophlegmatic growths.

[English]

(g) To Mrs. Christian 7 August, 1746.

Dear Mad^{m}

Since I had ye pleasure of seeing you I have looked over such Memorandums as I had relating to y^{r} Case, and I have also, with great care, considered the present state of y^{r} disorder. I find that I can now safely venture to prescribe some Antihysteric Nervous and corroborating Remedies wch I was obliged formerly to omitt apprehending that they might prove too forcing. As there is not now the same cause to abstain from them I hope that they may be of considerable service to you for the above-mentioned purposes and that you will also find them good against Wind, and moderately restringent. I dare not direct medicines that are more restring^{t} until I am certain that the redundant humours are carried off by a free and regular insensible perspiration, wch the present remedies are intended to promote. If I shd not have an opportunity of calling at Unerigg before you have finished these Remedies I hope you will be so good as to let me know how they agree with you, and whether you find any alteration from them. I shall take care to send you further directions about them.

In regard to y^{r} way of living I cannot advise any alteration from wch I could hope for Advantage.

My Spouse joins in our Compliments to you and your family. We were greatly obliged to some of them for the favours they lately did us, and wish they could have afforded us more of their Company, than wch none could be more agreeable.

I am

(h) Mrs. Christian 7 August 1746

Electuary of powdered myrrh 3 scruples; Powdered gum mastic 1 scruple; British saffron powdered 2 scruples; Best castor 1 scruple; Gentian extract 2 scruples; [Deleted—Crocus martis astringent]. Oil of juniper 20 drops; Mechoacan syrup. Make up very accurately pills of 5 gr. Take 4 at 11 a.m. and 5 p.m. daily.
Take 4 spoonfuls of the infusion:
Flower of hypericum 1 scruples; Flower of camomile 1 scruple; Dried golden orange 1 scruple; Juniper berry a scruple. Cut, press out and divide the mixture into 6 papers. Take 1 paper in 1 pt. boiling water and drink like tea.[179]

[See Case No. 87]

Memoirs of Mrs. Milham's Case .

Spirit of sal ammoniac 1 ½ oz; Distilled sorrel 5 oz; Mix together and add: Mixture of soap liniment 1 ½ oz; Every night at bedtime rub the affected part by the growth with dry warm woollen cloths for quarter of an hour, then smear with the above mixture spread on woollen cloth.

For Mrs. Milham's white, cold, soft growth on her wrist.

[These are draft letters, to be sent out to other doctors, written in English.]

87 Mrs. Milham's Case.[180]

Mrs. J:M: a married Lady aged years, of a delicate Slender make, and naturally, but of a weak, infirm Constitution; by the Mother descended from a family much afflicted with Strumous Symptomes to which she her self seems rather disposed; a considerable white, Slugish Tumour, having lately appeared a little above the joynt of the Wrist,
Diseases which have preceeded, omitted

[179] Mrs. Christian was obviously a most important patient of Brownrigg. These notes, collected over a seven-year period of her illness, and here placed in the correct order, testify to that and other items, viz: she was obviously capable of accurately setting down her own initial symptoms in the letter sent to Dr. Mead, although, from professional etiquette, Mead replies to her own doctor, Clementson; Brownrigg was brought in as a third source of consultation; as she was an educated woman, Brownrigg was able to discuss in detail her own case with her, using fairly technical terms. The variety of treatments, and especially the use of expensive wines, show her social position as a member of the two leading families in Maryport; from Brownrigg's letters to her, it seems that they also met on a social basis; these are all fairly rough notes, with many amendments and scorings-out (these have been omitted in most cases for the sake of clarity).

[180] Mrs. Milham was Elizabeth Gale before marriage, and came from one of the most important families in Whitehaven.

At present she complains of an acute, fixed and continual Pain in the small of the Back; which sometimes affects the left Thigh, particularly the external part, from the great Trochanter downwards to the Articulation of the Knee occasioning a most violent shooting pain, inability to Motion, with a little Redness and Swelling 'tho not considerable. Her appetite is much impaired, with a daily loss of Strength, and Consumption of the Muscular part, and usualy, towards the Evening, an Exacerbation of these Symptomes, with great heat, Thirst and a soft quick pulse is observable; which continue till early in the Morning, when they go off by large colliquative Sweats. Her Respiration is quite free and easy, without Stitches or Narrowness of the Breath, 'tho she has now and then, a short dry cough, but which is not very troublesome. Neither does her Urine discover the least sign of any distemperature in the Uropoietick Organs, being natural as to quantite and qualitie. No Hysterical Symptoms. Complexion set retains fine, vivid Tongue. She has now passed two Periods without the benefit of the Menstrual fluxes, 'tho there is no reason to presume her being pregnant.

Mrs. Milham, a Gentlewoman about 22 years old born of a Father weak and tender & afflicted wth and died of A at years of age. Her mothers Relations have many of them been troubled wth Strumous Swellings and is herself exceeding fat and unwieldy and troubled with something like ye Gout, she married at and had Children before she was all of which died young except the Gentlewoman whose Case we are about to describe.

Of a very fair Complexion, fine skin and in every other respect extreamly beautifull but having of a very weak Constitution & exceeding tender & delicate having been always educated in a most indulgent manner, and easily affected from the least error in her way of living—but had allways never been afflicted with any remarkab. Illness. Tis almost 4 years since she was married she enjoyed a tolerable good state of Health till about a year after marriage when she fell with Child but then during the time she went with Child was often afflicted with a very violent pain in her Back wch was not relieved. Strengthening plaisters or any other external applications about the end of the 7th month of going with Child, she was seized with a very acute Inflamation of the Intestines wch was caused by Bleeding and other Antiphlogistick Remedies but left her in a very weak Condition. wch might be the reason that she was brought to bed about the end of the 8th month. She recovered but very slowly for a long time after delivery having a bad Appetite being very weak and much afflicted with the old pain.

Memoirs of Mrs. Milham's Case. but was by degrees restored to a good state of Health after the use of Testaceous Powders with Ipecac Diatrag. mixed in Milk, Spa Waters and a Bitter Infusion with Root of Stypt. Helv: & regular diet. Soon after delivery there appeared a Swelling on the outside of the Tibia about the middle of the right leg, it was soft, lax and indolent and discovered no signs of inflamation it continued for about 4 months rather growing a little red and painful. The Surgeon applied to it a Poultice wth White Lilly Roots & afterwards a Plaister of Galbanus wch entirely dispersed the swelling, instead of bringing it to Suppuration as the Surgeon expected. She then enjoyed a good state of Health till falling with Child for a second time & was afflicted with the Pain in her back more than ever especially w^n^ pritty far advanced in her Pregnancy, she was brought to bed the 2nd time about February last, whilst she lay in she was twice or thrice seized with violent Pains about the Stomach & Bowels without any great Thirst or fever and she had several blackish Stools, Emollient Clysters & other aperient Remedies were used in order to evacuate certain acrid Atrabilarious Humours wch were conjectured to occasion the Pains after a sufficient use of these opening Remedies.

This Gent. was married when 19 and the first after wherewith we know her afflicted was a violent Pain in the Loins wch seized her about 3 years ago about ye 5th Month when going with her first Child, and was not relieved by Strengthening Plaisters and other external Applications.[181]

The Elect. with the addition of a Besides the Symptoms above enumerated since we have attended her this last time she hath been much afflicted with the Pain in her Loins it comes on then goes off without any known Cause, some times continues three or four days together, and then is easing again for several days. It forces her to lye in Bed & Cannot move without great pain w^{n} it is very violent. She can scarcely walk, goes almost double, and of late she has discovered her Body to be much inclined to the right side, wch seems to proceed from the curve position in the Vertbra of the Loins, she perceived this crookedness first in the last Spring but it grew better upon recovering her Strength. The Pain seems seated pretty near the Os Sacrum, she says it goes does not occasion any sickness or Vomiting Neither does her Urine discover any distemperature in the Urinary Organs. About a fortnight ago she was also much disturbed with a very acute pain in the left thigh wch affected the wch seems to weaken her the most of anything. The Sweatings have of times been very moderate but have constantly returned upon a troublesome Night or two of the Pain; Her pulse is always regular but generally too quick towards the Evening, at wch times she has usually a Thirst. She has but a very bad Apetite for food, her Legs sometimes swell toward of Evening. Her strength is greatly impaired and a daily consumption of the Muscular parts is very observable. Her Respiration is quite short. She was, however by these Disorders and by Childbearing much emaciated reduced to very great weakness, her appetite was almost entirely gone and every morning she had most profuse sweatings. (The Pains in the back were of times excessive). For these Complaints the following Decoctions of the Bark mixed with several Bitter Ingredients were prescribed to be taken 3 or 4 times a day with some drops of Elixir of Vitriol: she afterwards took Spa Waters with Testaceous Powders and Milk as formerly only there remained in the right arm resembling a white lax indolent swelling; there also appeared about this time a white soft swelling on her right Elbow, not accompanied with any Pain, wch by degrees fell downwards to the Malleus externus where it fixed and still continues being extended upwards along the Radius from the extremity for a mere hand Breadth (2 inches) & Plaisters of Galbanum with powder of Pepper or very penetrating Saponaceous & alternating resolving Liniments.

By the use of wch remedies together with light and nourishing diet and riding and the advantage of the Summer Season in a Country Air her disorders (Pains and sweatings) were removed and she again recovered her Stomach & Strength. She had enjoyed an indifferent state of Health all the Summer and the Menses wch had not appeared after Childbirth for the first time since her Labour appeared about and again flowed in June and continued regular in July and August and only in smaller quantities than Usual but to

[181] This paragraph was a later addition.

recompence that she had also an irregular evacuation of Blood wch probably flowed from the too much debilitated Hemorrhoedal Vessels generally appearing after Stools. But about 6th September during the course of ye Menses, she exposed herself too much to the cold by riding a long Journey on a very cold and rainy day to wch she had seldom been accustomed—in a day or two after she perceived herself much altered for the Worse she was sometimes chill at other times had feverish Heats, and every Morning very profuse and weakening Sweatings, and appetite quite impaired, the Menses did not flow at the usual period, and have not since appeared, her strength was every day impaired and she found

Was called after she had been in this Condition—
Indications of cure
Answered by w^{ch}
Effects—Lumbago & Crookedness—
Other Corroborant Effects—Pain & Swelling in her Thigh—Lumbago
Profuse Sweating—Prostration of appetite
Glad to be more fully informed of the Nature of the Pain— and directed in Remedies

> Conserve of orange peel 1 oz; Conserve of wormwood 6 scruples; Catechu 2 scruples; Astringent crocus martis 1 oz; Powdered sugar 1 oz; Myrrh size of toasted nutmeg; Spec. diamber; Sugar and lemon syrup.
>
> Bark of red sandalwood 4 scruples; Cinnamon 1½ scruples; Orange peel ½ oz; Gentian root 1 oz; Aromatic camomile 1 oz; Zedoar 1 oz; Cardamom seeds 2 oz; Century 20 pecks; Wormwood 20 pecks; Salvia. Boil in spring water to 2 pts, strain and add: Liquid wormwood 1½ scruples; Tincture of Stypt. Helv. 1½ scruples; Lavender spirit 1 spoonful.

[Small page insert written in Brownrigg's neatest handwriting.]

The purpose intentions in the Cure of this Disease have been to assist the Digestion, Concoction and Assimulation of the Food, to Strengthen the Vessels, and keep under the febrile Paroxisms; to answer which she had been kept to a Diet of Meats of good Nourishment, and early digestion, particularly Milk with the Testaceous Powders. Internal remedies have been taken from the most efficaceous of the restringents, Corroborative of Stomatick Elapses; amongst which the Cortex has been tryed under Various Forms of preperations, but without the least good Success . . .

[English]

Dr. Mead and Dr. Lawson's Answer to a Description of Mrs. Milham's Case.

Sir,

I am very much obliged to you for your esteem and the opportunity you gave me of conferring with Doct^{r} Mead, who of all the Gentlemen I have had the good fortune to become acquainted with since my return to England I profess to esteem the most; his universal good character in all capacitys of life being totally confirmed by his private one has so much captivated me that I am exceedingly pleased to be entirely devoted to him.

After having perused with a great deal of attention your accurate description of Mrs. Milhams indisposition, I early on Wednesday morning waited on Dr. Mead with it, who after having maturely weighed the whole Case was of opinion with me that the chief disorder of your patient is an hereditary weakness so readily manifesting itself on the least error in the Non-Naturals, and also an obstruction in the glandular System.

In order to obviate which as far as it is possible we would recommend the medicines prescribed on the other Page. The Powders we hope will correct the praeternatural disposition of the Glands, and considerably contribute to remove their Obstructions; the Bolus to be taken every fourth or fifth day, or as you will see occasion, and also its dose to be augmented or moderated according to the condition your Patient is in, which is intirely left to your Prudence, we conceive will be serviceable in evacuating the faeces, corroborating the Stomach and Intestines, and thereby procure a proper Digestion and Concoction of the food, besides the carrying of the Propensity to a diarrhoea. The Haustus at night will allay the Febricula and Thirst that obtains at that time; and from the whole we hope the weakning sweats will cease and your Patient gain Strength as far as her delicate frame will admit of. We would further recommend, which we see you have already prudently done, that the food administered be of an easy digestion, and rather of a dryer than a liquid nature, for drink Bristol Water with a very little red Wine, moderate exercise and Air, in regard to heat and cold, and every evening and morning to have the Leggs and feet rubbed gently with dry Flannels.

Since the Cortex does not agree with the Lady in any Shape we are of Opinion it should not be tryed any more.

Doct^r Mead joins with me in our humble Service to yourself and Doct^r Dixon.

I very sincerely am Sir

Your most Obedient Servant,

London, 20 November 1740. Isaac Lawson.

For Mrs. Milham

Take a sponge burnt to blackness in a crucible 1 scruple; Powdered red coral ½ scruple; Powdered cinnamon 4 gr; White sugar 4 gr. Pound together and take in the morning & at 5 p.m. Laxative 4 oz—mix with equal parts water and cow's milk.
Powdered rhubarb 1 scruple.
Confection of Alkermes, make a pill to take first thing in the morning every 4th or 5th hour every day for revival.

Alkaline milky water ½ oz; Strong cinnamon ½ oz;
Powdered crabs eyes) each 14 gr.
Refined nitre)
Wild poppy syrup 1 scruple;
Make a draught. Take it every night as above.

R. M. I. L.

[Latin]

88 Consultation for Mrs. Sharp.

For six whole months now Mrs. Sharp has been troubled with a melancholy verging on mania. Her native temperament, even a hereditary disposition, has perhaps given this misfortune a handle. Indeed the father (of this gentlewoman) suffered for most of his life from intensely wild manias, but on top of this hereditary condition there were also other causes stirring up this affliction. In fact, she had long been affected by a very serious depression and after her last confinement nine months ago, her lochia flowed only very little and the almost complete suppression of her periods followed, which has endured stubbornly to this time.

Her doctor was summoned and in vain tried to stem the disorder with great bloodletting and frequent antimonic vomitories, with an electuary from native cinnabar, camphor, black hellebore, salad burnet, orange flavoured conserve and other melting ingredients. I should rather advise remedies for eliminating the heavy and stagnant humours, opening up the blocked, soft abdominal vessels, bringing out the suppressed menses, removing the lack of tone or spastic strictures which derive from an artery or the nervous system and finally to drive the excessive wild violent humours from the brain. All these seem more suitable.

Medicaments moreover of such a kind as soaps and gums of giant fennel and aloes mixed, aperient decoctions, foot baths and rubbing of the abdomen and the extremities should be long and constantly used. She has very humbly submitted all this to the judgment of expert doctors, whose help she may need in her travels.

Written Whitehaven, W. B.
7 December, 1740.

[English]

To Eld: Curwen Esqr.[182]

I was favoured with yo^{rs} by the last post and am much rejoyced to find that your old pain hath quite left you. Pursuant to some directions which I rec^{d} from Mrs. Curwen, I here send inclosed a short description of Mast^{r} Curwen's disorder; there are several Circumstances which I thought less material, and have therefore omitted them, as Mast^{r} having used the Cold Bath, etc. but with these particulars you may yourself acquaint those Physicians whom you shall think proper to consult. I sh^{d} be glad to know their sentiments about these. As to the Bath it may be looked upon as a kind of last resort, but perhaps may not be thought so in present Case altogether necessary, as Mast^{r} Curwen has no Swelling nor Stiffness nor pain remaining in his joints. As the Spring Season is now coming and I hope we need not fear any sudden return of the disorder & if Mast^{r} Curwen could be persuaded to refrain from violent Exercise, all other precautions would perhaps be less necessary.

I am
Yo^{r} much obliged
& most faithfull Servt.
W. B.

4th Feb: 1741.

[182] Eldred Curwen of Workington Hall was MP for Cockermouth in the 1730s and also High Sheriff for Cumberland.

[Small pages inserted, written in English.]

89 Mast^{r} Curwen[183] aged 12 years of a pretty robust Constitution, fine florid Complexion, and very active and allways enjoyed a good state of health, untill he was seized with the Rheumatism about three years ago. That disorder is not hereditary and came upon him and seized him as far as I can learn soon after he had violently heated himself by running, and then lying suddenly down upon the Ground and fallen asleep where he continued for several hours untill in which condition he was found and carried home in the dark night after a strict search made for him. Having been bled thrice and several remedies applied he recovered very well, and recovered perfectly free from any symptoms that had no return of that disorder before November last, when it again came upon him after catching cold by using violent exercise. In this second fit, I attended him, the pains were very violent, he was bled twice, and took Manna and Clysters to keep his body open, and drank large quantities of weak, small diluting Liquors but could scarce be persuaded to use any other internal remedies but by this method recovered pretty well in a fortnights time, only a dry Cough remained for about a week longer. But he had the most severe attack in January last for on the 6th day he heated himself very much playing violently at foot.ball & the same day in the evening found himself indisposed, and complained of flying Pains; on the 7th & 9th he grew more uneasy & his pains were very troublesome especially in his side and about the Breast, on the 10th, 11th and 12th his pains increased to a great degree, but seemed to fix more in his extremities he had used a proper diet but no other application was hitherto made. On the 13th I was called and found that the Pains had affected both feet especially the joints wch were then much swelled upon wch the pains abated, as they constantly did after this fit began he also complained of pains in his Wrists and fingers and frequently of pains in his Breast and Neck but seemed to be then most tormented by pains in his Shoulders wch were so very great that he could not help crying out continually day and night, and altho he could scarce move a leg yet was so exceedingly restless that he could not remain two minutes in any one posture but was constantly desiring to be removed.

The pains were attended with an especially acute Fever. He was very hot, and dry, his pulse exceeding and hard but regular, his Tongue dry and White, clear and high coloured, and had a great thirst, very costive in his body and moderately ordered about 10 oz of blood to be taken by Arm which was exceeding sizey and had little or no Serum.

The fever was so very violent I prescribed anti-phlogistic decoctions of the Aperient Roots with Nitrous salts dissolved in them wch with persuasion of Mrs. Curwen he took very carefully, his Body was also kept open with emollient Clysters, he used a very low diet and drank plentifully of thin diluting liquid made warm. The 15th I saw him again the pains were then almost as acute as the 13th and had continued so very severe in almost all parts of his body without any considerable intermission but abating w^{h} they had begun to swell, but as his fever was nearly abated and his urine deposited a sediment I did not think fit to bleed him and ordered him to persist in the use of the remedies.

In the Afternoon he broke out into a breathing sweat, and the pains abated and he slept.

[183] Master Curwen, son of Eldred Curwen of Workington (1692–1745) a landowner and rival to Sir James Lowther in the coal trade.

In ye 17th in the Evening I found his skin very moist and his pains almost quite gone. And when I saw him on the 21st, he was so well that he had got down Stairs, and had a tolerable good appetite, he was quite free from the fever and had no Cough, nor no stiffness nor swelling nor Pain remaining in his Limbs, & hath continued well ever since. The other fits of ye Rheumatism he had before were much like this, wch I have here described, but not so severe.

In order to prevent any return of the Disorder I advised that he might be kept warm clothed. That he would carefully abstain from all violent Exercise and be very cautious no way to expose himself to catch of cold, and to use a light Diet of Milk and Vegetables for breakfast & Supper. I also prescribed the following decoction wch he now used

For Mast^{r} Curwen.

> Guaiacum shavings 2 oz; Red sandalwood shavings 3 scruples; Chopped currants 1½ oz; Wormwood salts ½ scruple. Boil for ½ hour in river water. Make up 2 pts. After boiling add:
> Sassafras wood shavings ½ oz; Liquorice root 1 oz; Orange juice 1½ scruples; Strain and add:
> Strong cinnamon water 1½ oz;
> Drink 5 spoonfuls of this warm in a single dose at dawn and at night.

90 Mr. Christian commonly called Major Christian,[184] a man of 64 formerly given to wine and excessive drinking, affected for many years by his kidneys. Last November after taking a chill he developed a troublesome stiffness in the Lumbar Region, then in one hand then the other. Lastly on 5th September passed bloody urine and grumae of blood once and the same again in 8 days. Almost continuous strangury. No appetite for meat. Presented natural bowel movements.

[The above is on a small piece of paper, pasted in the Casebook above the following in English:]

Our diagnosis for Mr. Christian of the Isle of Man.
Whitehaven, 27 May 1741.

Sir,

I hope that your friend has given me so full and just account of your disorder, that from this description, I shall be able to form a right judgment concerning it, I observe what he relates of your having formerly, for several years, been subject to the gravell & Nephritick complaints and of your having for six months past been much afflicted with violent pains about your back and loins, and having attentively considered these severall circumstances, and compared 'em with your present complaints, am induced to believe that some stone or stones, which have for a long time been lodged in the kidnies, and are too large to pass thro the ureters into the bladder, are the cause of your present disorders and which by

[184] Major Christian was a relative of the Christians of Unerigg and may have had his symptoms written to Brownrigg on the recommendation of his relatives.

Lacerating the Kidnies and opening the vessels, occasion the violent pains, the discharge of bloody urine and grumous globs of blood, strangury and the other Symptomes wherewith you are now so very much afflicted.

In Such a Case it would be highly improper to attempt to expell the stones into the bladder by stimulating and forcing remedies, or to endeavour to disolve them by Mrs Stephen's Medicines, or other Lithotripticks, all therefore that can rationally be proposed, is, to prevent the pain and Laceration which the stones occasion, to heal and strengthen the vessels of the kidnies, and so remove the strangury bloody urine, and the rest of the Symptoms, which being effected you may a long time bear the stones in this present situation without any considerable inconveniency. In order therefore to answer these several intentions of cure, and to remove the present symptoms, it will be necessary that you should carefully pursue the following method:

Diet.

Let your food be of such kinds of food as are light and easy of digestion, viz, for breakfasts and suppers make use of broths, gruels, and especially milk if it agree with you. You may also take tea or chocolate in morning if you chuse them: for your dinner take chicken veal or any other light kinds of meat, Spinnage, Mercury and all kinds of greens will be exceeding proper.

For your common drink use bristol water, or light river water with a toast in it, also a glass or two of good old port wine after dinner and Supper, and abstain from all kinds of malt drink or spiritous liquors. Go constantly warm cloathed, go early to bed at the nights, take care not to ride on a trotting horse or to use any violent motion, but gentle exercise or walking in the house or garden will be very serviceable. Take a gentle purge of Manna and the pulp of Casia once a week which must be prepared after the following manner.

Take a paper of the manna each of which contains an ounce and disolve it in a pint of whey made with Reanet when the Manna is disolved by warming them together, gently over the fire, then strain the Liquor thro a linnen cloath, then disolve it in three quarters of an ounce of pulp of Casia by stirring them together. This quantity must be drunk of at three or four draughts early in the morning, in two hours time, and drink whey or posset drinks in the working. if it does not give you three or four stools you may augment the quantity both of the Manna and pulp of casia, as occasion requires—

On the days on which you do not take the purges take three of the pills thrice a day namely two hours after breakfast, 3 hours after dinner and going to rest, and after each dose of them, drink a small draught of new whey.

I cannot at present commend to you the use of Scarborough water, thinking it too stimulating and forcing, perhaps it may be more proper hereafter. It is impossible for me at this distance to advice as the various contingencies may require, but according to present appearances, I hope that this method may agree with you very well, and that by pursuing it five or six weeks the symptoms may be entirely removed. I sincerely wish you a perfect recovery of your health and am

Your most obed^t^ Servant,
W. Brownrigg.

The Pills I ordered were as follows:

For Major Christian

> Choice manna 1 oz; Take 6 papers of these. Pulped cassia root 6 oz; Root of choicest rhubarb 1½ scruples; Powdered mastic 1 oz; Saffron 1 scruple; Catechu 1½ scruples; Liquid extract of liquorice ½ oz; Strasbourg turpentine. Make hard pills of equal size, each one 1 drachm. Make 10 pills.

[The following consultation copy letters were written in Latin in at least 2 different hands, neither of them Brownrigg's.]

To Mynheer the esteemed J. Van Swieten, M.D., at Leyden, Holland.

Most esteemed sir,

Pardon me for wishing to offer for your judgment the following case. You may not know me by sight, but your learning and powers are not hidden from me, ever since I applied myself to medical studies as a student at your famous university. Therefore I am easily persuaded to seek your counsel in a case of such importance to me, and I strongly ask you to reveal it to me. The case is as follows.

W. C., a man of between 50 and 60 years old, of a rather robust and stout nature of body of medium height, rarely eating or drinking to excess, attends quite diligently to exercises by riding and walking. He was formerly accustomed to the best of health, but he passed gravel. Pains appeared and a rheumatism now wandering over his limbs like Lumbago afflicted him. For two and a half years he was troubled with a frequent obstructed bowel and then, until his bowel cleared, he noted the first part of the excrement to be streaked with blood. Since in fact he observed no illness or bad humours between the evacuations nor was ever infirm, he thought little of this passage of blood. In the month of August 1739 he was confined to bed with an irregular fever of a quite nervous nature, with very great sweatings, his spirit and pulse lowered and he had disturbances in the head. These lasted for a month and more. They continued with almost the same manner and finally, without an obvious crisis, they were dissipated after the use of dilutants and aperient medicines dissolved in salt water.

[The following page is blank, so there may have been more case details not copied in.]

[English]

Kendal. December 18, 1741.

Dr Sir,

Yours I have had some time by me, and delayed answering it till I could also send you Short, but as that is at Carlisle, and I don't know when I may expect it I would no longer differ given you the answer. I had from the several Gentlemen, I consulted on my father's case; I leave you to make your own observations on 'em, but must confess I found nothing in any of them to make me change my first sentiments of the cause of the disease, which I glad to find agreed exactly with that you gave me In yours, and which you will find us supported in by Dr. Swieten: I hope the Gentlemen at Ed[r] carry it too far in giving it the Tumour the appellation of cancrodes, and would Gladly flatter myself by having this hope confirmed by the event, from the great ease my father had found in adhearing to his elect: ex Ethiop Miner. et Cort. Borav, & the aq. Calcis, both to wash down the Elect: ex Aethiop: and as his constant drink, he is now able to pass his nights without Laudanum which for some time he was obliged to have recourse to, tho he never exceeded 15 grains. I can not send you D[r] Boswels letter, but I shall give you an extract of it so far as relates to this case, he says, he had consulted with some of the most famed and experienced of the Faculty with them, and was sorry to tell me they were of the opinion, it was a Scirilius of the worst kind In the Rectum, or neck of the Bladder and were afraid it would be deadly, that a Gentleman told him he lost three patients last winter by that ailment, he found Glysters of Decot: Capit. Papav: alb, in aq. Calc: cum ob: Lini et Pearls Luceat to Give ease for sometime, and that an Elect: ex Cort. Peru: et Aethiop: miner: seemed to perlong life, without adding to the pain he gave opiates to make the nights easy. In short says he treat your Patient as Incurable, but whose life may be perlonged, and made easier by avoiding every thing that may encrease the Cancerous disposition of the Tumor, This you see agreed pretty much with Mr. Monrow.

[English]

Dumfries June 18, 1741.

D[r] Doct[r]

This night I had yours, and being to go out of Town in the morning, I shall have just as much time as to write an answer to the most urgent part of it, as which will I hope excuse what may be defective in the matter as well as that I have not writ in your Language.

The Gentlemans case appears to be plain, a tumor in the Rectum, but shall not pretend to say whether it may bear the consequence of his fever, or from the Hemorrhoids, or whether it is of a benign or of a Bad kind, a simple tumor in that part is sufficient to produce all the uneasy Symptoms of Tenesmus and strangury and the blood may be either from the Tumor or erosion of the intestine, and continual severe reeding, it is not competent for me to judge of these things at a distance no more than of the patients constitutions, whether he Labours under any particular discrasy, upon all which a prognostick is to be formed. Tho he has higherto kept up both in his habits and appetite, I am affraid he may soon feel himself languishing by the continual pain and anguish he suffers as well as discouragement, as well as loss of blood which in an advanced age must wear the habit first and he begins to be sensible of this in a good degree.

As the seat of the Desease may be easily come at you must treat it much after the Chirurgical ways by making proper applications with judgement and caution till the nature of the thing is discovered. Injections ought to be used frequently, especially going to Bed that they may be retained, these Injections may be made of what we call here wades Balsam or the Balls paralitick Calcei: taken down with Rosar water, plantain, elderflower and calcium adding opium and egg yolk: more or fewer of these may enter into the composition according as the pain bleeding or signs of Orosion shall require, so as they may be more or less astringent, discutient Erient anodine, everything must be avoided that can give irritation for fear of increasing pain and fluxion, the pain and weakness of the back may be relieved by wearing constantly a plaister of vegetable juices with gum of which is better than the mercuriale, with some alom, crocus, Camphire added to it, renewing it frequently, it should cover all the os coccygis, this is the only way that appears to me to reach the disease in the very part affected. If a cacochymick or Scorbutick habit, this Must be alleviated by an appropriated course, either of milk or whey or mineal waters, perhaps Moffat, and all methods should be fallen upon to keep the animal parts in good plight, by doing everything; That will keep up the appetite promote digestion and procure a constant supply of good wholesome nourishment which is the best way to men a set of bad juices, where a stomakick balsomak elixir of myrrh, sugar, extract of gentian: fort auriant; digested in Canary, should be given immediately before or after meals, thrice a day in any ordinary drink, whatever is taken by the mouth can have no effect immediate upon the place affected except purgative to cleanse the bowels, but must be intended in some shape to mend the habit upon the footing of antiscorbuticks, an Electuary of sulphide of mercury or powdered potash made up with orange conserve and syrup might be given a morsel twice a day, with a mild decoction of the woods, or Bate's water, the morning dose may be taken two hours before he rises to promote a breathing fit, I do not what mercurials have been used but if they be not very mild of the Ethiops or Cinnabar kind, they will wear him much, nor do I think that purgatives stronger than Manna, oil, cream of tartar, Rhubarb & the like perhaps the flowers of Sulphur solution or Linctus, with these might be a good effect to keep the Belly open which should always be consulted, this is all that occurs to me at present both against an ill diet and costiveness, if you favour me hereafter which I shall be glad off. with a further correspondence upon this head I shall endeavour to make up or correct what ever shall be awanting or amiss in this, I guess who this friend of yours is, and if I could at any time or in any manner be of use to you or him You might make use of me as your own But for all my hurry I must give you joy, and may you in this new state long enjoy plenty and contentedness of mind.

You may believe me your Eben Gilchrist.[185]

D^r^ S^r^

I had the favour of yours the 15 Instant and after a Serious perusial of It Its scarce possible to say much up on it. the cause is most distincly fully related and the method of cure has been very judiciously followed out I am wholy of opinion that some large Branch of the Haimeroehdall Vean is Ruptured which is the occasion of the flux of Blood to be so frequent and particularly so great quantities of the fesces being hardened and I am aprehensive there is a stone of no small size in the Bladder which you may be easily satisfied of by sounding. to remove all which complaints I should think a mass of Saponaceous pills with some Emulient Decoction Infusion wil be of great use in order to keep an open Belly and every second or third night an Injection of Some Balsamick ingredient to be given in such a way, and to keep the same all night, and to use a nourishing dyet of such foods as yields the smaller quantities of fesces. To abstain from all kinds of malt Liquors, and no wine but purely for a cordial to support the spirits. to use little or no excercise til you are satisfied that the mouths of Blood vestels are stped, and walk when obliged but slowely, as I don't doubt of your having the advice of every able phicisians I

[185] Ebeneezer Gilchrist (1707–74), author of 'An essay on nevous fevers', *Medical Essays and Observations*, Edinburgh, T. & W. Ruddimans, 1737, vol. 4, pp. 347–406.

shall not be too tedious up on you you have upon the other side a formula of all the pills and decoctions which you may use either to add or take from it what seems unnecesary I wish my good and worthy friend a speedy recovery, and to you all manner of happin[s] be so good as to Lett me hear from you as soon as you have made tryal of this or any other methods of cure

I am with all due esteemd D[r] D[r] your most obed: hum: servt: Jno. Hay.

Dumf., June 24
1741

[English]

S[r]

I am much afraid your Father's symptoms are owing to a Tumor of a bad kind, which surrounds the Rectum, at that place where the stricture of Contraction is, the small pendulous Tubercles coud not produce so much disorder, whereas a Schirrhous or steatomateous Tumor in that part will account for all appearances. I have had several Patients with such Tumors, in that part as I imagine your father, my old friend to have, none of them were cured, every thing that irritated did harm, by keeping the Bellies of the patients loose with the milder laiture, they were Less pained and less plaged with the Tenesmus, Emolient pultices externally aplied to the pireneum made them some easier. In two such patients a Large Suppuration formed near the Anus, while the supuration went on, they were in racking pain. After the mater was discharged they were much more free of the pain then before it happened, but were not freed by this discharge under which they slowly died, those who had no Supuration, had the advantage of Dying sooner you see I have a very unfavourable opinion of this case, and tho I have not proposed any cure, I have hinted at what may give some mitigation of the pain and Tenesmus, which I do not think the extirpation of the pendulous Tumors will do.

I am very glad of hearing of your welfare and will most willingly serve you, when occasion offers.

Your most obed[t] Serv[t]
Alex : Monro

Ednr : Sep[tr] 29
1741

[The above consultations sought from Van Swieten, a doctor at Kendal, Dr. Gilcrest in Dumfries, Dr. Hay in Dumfries, and Dr. Monro were all giving opinions on Brownrigg's father, who did not actually die until 1760.]

[Written in Latin, but still in a different handwriting to Brownrigg's.]

To the most learned, most expert doctor, and most eminent George Carlyle.
G. Van Swieten sends his greetings.

I have endeavoured with the greatest possible attention to consider the case you very precisely described, and after weighing everything carefully, I have come to this opinion.

Two and a half years ago I saw a constriction of the bowel with hard faeces adhering to the intestine, with the result that this began to be forced open by the pressure, while the hard excrement passed through and were everywhere smeared with bloody streaks. The trouble increased further by the veins swelling and making the obstruction worse and it narrowed the channel of the intestine and produced tenesmus. For all that which by its weight or sharpness irritates the lower intestine, its lower surface makes the bowel and channel of deposition. Then the swelling of the dilated vessels seems to occupy that area which lies next to the colon or the bladder, and then more or less turns its bad blood or tenesmus to the intestine or bladder. There seems to me, from a diagnosis of the rest of the symptoms, to be a fairly clear reason. I see a difficult cure as far as my prognosis is concerned. Already very many excellent remedies have been tried, but the patient's generally good disposition and his healthy appetite give him hope. The following will be of assistance in a cure. The bowel cleared out once a day for three days with a gentle clyster or scrape. Thereafter you must make use of a diet whereby no, or almost no faeces are accumulated in the intestines. It would be very good if he could live on meat broth alone. Take 4 times a day one twelfth of hot decoction B. The following will procure relief for all parts affected by tenesmus and strangury. At the same time it produces less improvement in the vessels. On alternate days after, clear the bowel with one 4 oz injection of warm decoction C, if there appears an ulcerans. I hope you will carefully note an improvement from these items. Farewell and have my best regards.

Written Holland, 26 October 1741.

A. Fine oil 4 ; Mercury & honey 2 oz; Barley water. Make up a clyster.

B. Marshmallow root; Mallow leaves 3 oz. Boil for 1 hour in spring water, strain, then add
Mullein 1 oz; Liquorice 3 oz; Mineral oil. Boil in a sealed container for ¼ hour, strain and add 4 oz chicory oil.

C. Root of pentaply 3 ; Bistort 3 oz; Tormentil 3 oz; Boil for 1 hour in water; add red rose petals 6 after 1 boiling only. stand for ¼ hour then add 16 drops of olive oil. Repeat the dose once.

91 Mrs. Jolson of Cockermouth, a married woman of 50 or over, and in 1741 at the beginning of spring she was seized with a shivering, with a small fever, then an erysipelatic swelling appeared on her face. Then an almost identical swelling seized one leg, accompanied by pain and considerable heat. When the inflammation went, the whole leg was affected by a leucophlegmatic tumour. I prescribed venesection and purging and when the inflammation went I prescribed small beer and riding, by which she felt considerable alleviation.

Guaiacum wood shavings ½ lb; Root of fresh oak fern 6 oz; Root of oxylapath 4 oz; Root of monks' rhubarb 4 oz. Boil this in fresh beer instead of hops. Reduce 5 measures to 4 in the beer, strain and after fermenting in the flask, suspend in the cask a small bag with the following ingredients, then drink about ½–1 pt of this beer every morning and at 5 p.m. While using this, if the belly does not respond twice a day, take Pill Ruffi of 4 or 5 grams when going to sleep. Cochineal leaves 4 pecks; Agrimony leaves 2 pecks; Salvia leaves 2 pecks; Roman wormwood 2 pecks; Dried dandelion root ½ lb; Seed of sweet fennel 1½ oz. Mix the ingredients in a little bag.

In the month of July 1742, after a shivering fit, she had the same swelling occupying her face and head, accompanied by fever and thirst. I prescribed firstly powdered nitrates and shells, and on every third day an antiphlogistic purge made from Glauber's Salt, manna and similar provisions. This method removed the inflammation and I ordered the following:

Gum of myrrh 3 scruples; Sweet aloes 1 drachm; Saffron 2 drachms; Venetian soap 1½ scruples; Pure native turpentine 6 gr; Tincture of castor 10 drops; Juniper oil 10 drops. Measure accurately 4 pills of 1 drachm. Take 3 first thing in the morning and 1 every night at bed time with 4 oz of the following warm liquid.
Shavings of guaiacum bark 1½ oz; Shavings of red sandalwood 1 scruple; Sarsaparilla root 1 scruple; Fresh burberry 1½ oz; Crushed raisins 1 oz.
Boil for half an hour in spring water. Make up to 2 pts. Add: Fresh dandelion root 2 oz; Bark of sassafras ½ oz; Juniper berries 2 scruples; Pure nitre salt 2 scruples.

[Two small pages inserted.]

92 A. Mrs. Crackplace.

To remove the humours from the face, it helps by rubbing of the extremities with these items in spring water to remove the inflammation.

Very strong vinegar 8 oz; Savory 1 scruple; Tincture of benzoin ½ scruple; Spirit of camphor.

or, wild lettuce, a nutritive ointment.

Antiphlogistic remedies should be taken internally. They will also be evacuated by all these and natural nose blowings and gentle evacuant and corroborative remedies to be taken faithfully for a long time. As such I recommend the

Myrrh; saffron; rhubarb; liquorice extract; ammoniac, Pill Ruffi or aloes; Venetian turpentine. Take twice a day with a decoction of woods and nitrous roots.

Diet—whey and the like. Above all, her feet should be kept warm and all her body kept well covered.

Mental condition—by riding—and sound sleeps.

B. See Riverius, page 503. On a nobleman with frequent relapses of erysipelas cured completely by drinking mercury dissolved in wine. The cause was thought by Riverius to be strengthening by the wine of the expulsive faculty hence the material of erysipelas was removed by natural blowing of the nose. Paré uses this ointment for erysipelas:

Golden litharge ½ oz; Flower of benzoin ½ scruple; Camphor 1 drachm; Very strong vinegar 1 oz; Sweet almond oil 1½ oz.
Make a thick ointment. Smear a very little carefully on the face when going to bed. Lac virginis.
Dissolve the lethargics in distilled vinegar then pour in drops of oil of tartar.

Phlegmonoid erysipelas inflames the whole face very badly and also the head, particularly after incomplete and difficult periods, as described by Horstius *Works*, II, p. 112, also on p. 443.[186] One must abstain from fat, oily and spicy food as well as spirituous liquors.

[English]

93 To Jn° Christian Esqr at Unerigg[187] 4 Aug. 1742

Dear Sir

When I had last the pleasure of seeing you I made most diligent Inquiries concerning the Nature of your Constitution, your Manner of Living, and those complaints wherewith you had lately been affected.

Preface

I have since with the utmost attention considered the several particular circumstances which I then collected together, with a View to form a clear and certain Judgement of the Nature & Causes of your Late Disorder, and to prescribe such Methods as are most proper to be pursued in order to preserve your future Health.

Diagnosis of illness

From these particulars it evedently appears that the Disorder wherewith you were lately affected was a slight Resolution of certain Nerves, whereby the Organs of Speech became, for a short time, unfit to perform their proper Offices. a Chillness and Heaviness over all your Body, and some other Symptoms did also proceed from the same Cause by which the Nerves subservient to the Organs of Speech were thus affected.

Observations as the illness progressed.

Altho their Disorder was in itself very slight and easily gave way to Bleeding and other proper Remedies; yet I cannot but greatly approve of the desire you show of guarding as much as possible against any future attacks of it, since Distempers of this kind altho they may commonly be prevented, yet oftimes cannot be cured without the greatest difficulty.

Main causes of illness.

In order therefore rightly to prescribe such methods as may prevent any return of your late Distemper, it is necessary to weigh and consider the several Causes which might concurr in producing it.

Some Disposition to this Disorder might arise, partly from your Native Temperament, being such as Physicians call Sanguineo-phlegmatick, from your age, as you now begin to approach towards a time of Life when crude Pituitous and glutinous humours do naturally begin to abound in the blood, and often occasion the Gout & other Chronick Distempers; partly also from a Scorbutick Lentor wth which your Juices are slightly infected as appears

[186] Gregor Horst, *Opera medica*, 1661.
[187] Husband of Mrs. Christian, Case No. 86.

from the Spots upon your Leggs: but chiefly from your too sedentary, inactive and studious course of Life, joined to a full and nourishing Diet, by which means you are become too corpulent & unwieldy the perspirable matter is not evacuated in sufficient quantities; the solid parts of the Body are relaxed, and the fluids are in too large a quantity accumulated in the Vessels.

Immediate cause of illness.

This Habit of Body might be the remote cause of your Disorder, but the more immediate cause seems to have been a too great fullness and too sudden and violent Distention of the Arteries of the Brain & of its membranes; whereby the veins and sinusses of the Brain being compressed their Cavities were not proportionate to the quantity of Blood which ought to have circulated through them so that the free reflux of the Blood from the Brain was in some measure retarded. *By the same distended Arteries some of the Nervous Canals were intirely compressed, and consequently the Actions of those Nerves were for some time suspended.

*The too great thickness of the blood might also concurr in producing this its Stagnation.

That the Disorder was thus produced, several Circumstances which preceeded it leave no room for doubt. A day or two before you were seized, you were obliged to use more exercise & to live a little more freely than common; By wch means the Circulation must necessarily have been accelerated, and a more than usual quantity of Blood accumulated in the Vessels. On the Morning that the Disorder came upon you, You had heated yourself much with walking, which must have occasioned a still greater rarefaction & motion of the blood, and a more violent distention of the Vessels; in that condition you sat down to your Studies in a cool place, by wch means the external parts of y^{r} body became suddenly contracted whilst the fluids yet remaining in their rarefied state even were consequently propelled in too large quantities into those Vessels whose Tone was weaker towards the external parts, and especially towards the Brain which being on all sides surrounded with a firm and solid tone is not liable to suffer such Alterations in its dimensions, as other parts of the body, and when any of its Vessels are distended more than usual they must necessary compress others as they have ye Liberty to swell outwardly.

Indications for prophylaxis.

1. To prevent as much as possible a too great plenitude and fullness of the Vessels, and a too great accumulation of humours in the habit of Body.
2. To guard against all such Accidents as may any ways tend to occasion a too large & sudden motion of the Blood towards the Head & a too great Distention of the Vessels of the Brain.
3. To attentuate and dissolve the crude Lentors and Viscidity of the Blood, so that it may be thoroughly concocted, & the Nervous fluid secreted from it may be fit to pass through the minutest Cannals without any danger of obstructing them. I thought it proper thus freely and without reserve to communicate to a person of y^{r} precedence & knowledge, my Sentiments concerning the nature of y^{r} late disorder, and those intentions which ought to be answered in order to prevent any future attacks of it; hoping that if my reasonings should meet with your approbation, you would by them be induced more readily & exactly

to comply with such rules of living as the future preservation of your Health seems to me to require. To answer the several Preservatory Indications above mentioned I therefore recommend the following Method:

A curing diet.

Let your Diet be of such things as are easy of Digestion, & of good and light nourishment, so that they may not afford gross, heavy, & viscid Juices. There are few kinds of Food that you need intirely abstain from, alltho some kinds are greatly preferable to others. Roast meats are better than boiled; and boiled than such as are baked; Mutton, Beef, Fowls, Veal are to be preferr'd before Pork; White fish, before salmon & Trout; Beans, dried Pease, all Salt & dried Meats are worst of all.

Let your drink be rather strong, and in little quantities, than small, and in larger. For your common Draught at Victuals, Water mixt with about a fourth parts of good red Port is very proper, with a Glass or two of the same Wine; or of some good strong and light White wine, or sometimes a little Punch after dinner & Supper. Malt Liquors, especially mild soft Ale, I can by no means approve, as it is too apt to produce thick impure and viscoid juices, unfit to circulate through the minutest Vessels, and tends to create a too great fullness and Corpulency; perhaps also you may not be able so thoroughly to digest it now as you have been formerly. Tea will make a good Breakfast, but am affraid that if taken in the afternoons, it may relax the solids too much, and weaken the Tone of the Stomach, and put a check to perpiration. I recommend to you to continue the use of your Light Suppers; and think that the Times at wch you are accustomed to take y^{r} meals are the most proper.

You cannot go to bed or arise at more reasonable Hours than those you have been accustomed to. Only think that you should rather diminish than increase your time of sleeping & should endeavour to wean yourself from Sleep in the Afternoons. Exercise is a great and necessary preservative of Health in all ages and almost all Constitutions, without the pritty constant use of wch you can scarce preserve y^{r} self from Chronical Distemper. I therefore would advise you to walk about, especially in the forenoons, as much as you can without weariness, & to ride out every day in y^{r} Chaise. And by this means I hope in a little time, you will be able to ride on Horseback; wch exercise, would of all others, do you the greatest Service.

I also would advise you to be moderate in your Application to Business, And to abstain as much as possible from night Workings, or long and severe Studies. To close application to Study being apt to prevent the Digestion of the Food, and Concoction of the Humours, and to obstruct perspiration.

A Cheerfull and easy Disposition of mind will also greatly contribute towards preserving your Health. Frictions may be exceeding usefull, so that it would be very proper to rub yourself all over with a Flesh brush every night and morning. It will also be advisable to wash your Leggs and feet well in warm water once or twice a Week before you go to rest, and after they are dryed, to rub them well with a warm dry flannel. But this method should not be pursued if it occasions any swelling or Soreness of your Leggs. The Pills & Wine wch I have directed Mr. Clementson to prepare for you are chiefly designed to answer the first and third Indications by gently promoting all the natural Evacuations, Dissolving all viscid & glutinous Humours, and Strengthening the whole Body especially the Nervous System. I would advise you to continue the use of them for five or six Weeks.

These Rules w[ch] I have Mentioned I think the most material, in other things your own prudence will easily direct you. When I have an opportunity w[ch] I hope may be in a little Time I shall discourse wth you further upon these Subjects. If you are affraid that any Inconvenience might arise from a too sudden compliance with any of the Rules afore mentioned, I beg that you would do it by degrees, but with as much Speed as is consistent with your Health ease and Satisfaction. Since I have the greatest reason to hope that this Method if carefully pursued will with the Divine assistance affectually prevent any future return of y[r] late Disorder, and may also in other Respects contribute to preserve your Health. That you may long enjoy these Blessings is the most hearty prayr of

Y[r] most obliged Humble Serv[t]

W. B.

[Latin]

Mr. Potter of Cockermouth.

Dr. Askew's Advice in Mr. Potter's Case.

> Olibanum gum 2 scruples; Sacocolla gum 2 scruples; Gum mastic 2 scruples; Turpentine 2 scruples. Mix with hollyhock syrup and make up 12 pills, each one 1 scruple. Take 5 in the morning and evening every day for 6 weeks. Besides taking the above with 4 oz of tea made from the following:
> A young orange 1 peck; Water betony 1 peck; Brook lime 1 peck; Liquorice root 6 scruples. Squeeze the materials with ½ pt of tea in boiling water.
>
> Powdered crabs eyes 10 gr; Powdered shell of common crab 10 gr; Comfrey root 10 gr; Fine sugar ½ scruple. Make some powders and take every morning with 1 spoonful of ass's milk. Take ½ pt of that or in place of ass's milk use same quantity of barley water and cow's milk.

A. A.

Newcastle. April 28, 1741.

[English]

Sir,

I hope the Method here recommended will be of use to you and I should prefer Asses Milk to take of y[r] Thirst to Cow's Milk and Barley Water w[ch] are advised only as a Substitute if the other cannot well be got. Your Breakfast may be Chocolate, Rice, Gruel with a little red wine or a warm Gelly. Y[r] Dinner white meats or Puddings of Rice or Sago. Y[r] Supper Gruels of Sago or Rice or the like.

I am,

Yours, etc.

A. Askew.

Y[r] Common Drink to be red Wine and Bristol Water.

For Mr. Potter.

Repeat the prescribed pills of Sarcocolla gum and Olibanum. Take 5 every morning and 5 in the afternoon. Take the above decoction with 3 oz of Peruvian bark, balsam and quince. Drink red wine with Bristol Water for your common drink.

December 11, 1741. A. A.

[English]

Mr. Potter.

Sir,

I have carefully weighed all Circumstances of your Case and would advise you to use the Remedies here prescribed which I commend to you for the Cleansing, healing and strengthening quality which they exert chiefly upon the Urinary Organs, and hope that your Complaints may be intirely removed by these and such like Remedies if the use of them is sufficiently pursued. I greatly approve of the Diet already directed you by Dr. Askew and desire that you would continue the Use of it. The inclosed are Dr. Askew's prescriptions wch I recd from Mr. Simpson on Monday last, I should have wrote to you yesterday, had I not expected to have seen you today at Cockermouth; but I am obliged to put off my Visit to my friends there until the latter end of this week or the beginning of ye Next. At wch time I hope I shall be able to judge how the Remedies I now order you will agree with you, and shall give you such further directions as I shall find proper.

I desire my kind respects to y^{r} good Lady & Miss Potter and am with the most hearty wishes for y^{r} perfect Recovery.

S^{r} : y^{r} most Obed^{t} Humble Servt

W. B.

25 August 1741.

Gum mastic 3 scruples; Olibanum 1½ scruples; Rhubarb 1 scruple; Liquorice extract 2 scruples; Silvery turpentine. Make up a firm mass and make it into 12 pills of 1 drachm each. Take 4 at once at dawn and at night. Take an Infusion of tea—4 oz, sweetened with honey as your drink with them. Make up the tea as below:

It is made with St. John's wort—Yarrow—Leaves of scabious—Ground ivy—Brook lime—2 scruples of each. Gum Arabic 1½ scruples. Pulped juniper berries 2 scruples: make the infusion in 9 oz of boiling water.

[English]

Dr Sir,

This two days past Mr. Potter has had a Hecking Violent Vomiting upon him at times, which he vomits is nothing but Phlegm, & he Complains of a pain on his left side below his Rib's. He has no Stomach for Solids, nothing but Spoon Meats, & that is According to Dr. Askews Directions that he takes, he Complains off a pricking pain in his anus, in ye Morning he voids a quantity of Glutinous mater from ye Peernis before any water can pass, which gives me reason to believe there is some Ulcer form^{d} upon ye Prostate glands, & a great heat when he makes Water. Yesterday in ye Evening he Complained very much, but this Morning he finds him self much better, he seams very Desireous to have a gentle Vomit if you should think it proper, what he made this Morning I have sent it, but its glutinous Substance will be incorperated wth ye water, it is all the quantity he makes at a time. In haste

Your most Obed. & Humble
Servt to Command
John Simpson.

Dec. 1741.
Cockermth Thuesday
Morning.

P.S. If you return an answer please to send it to Thom^{s} Smith his partner who is now in Whitehaven at Mr. Potter^{s} Shop.

[English. Brownrigg's reply to Simpson, written on the back of the letter sent to him.]

Dear Sir,

From the Strangury Heat & Urine in Making Water, and evacuation of the said purulent Matter without any mixture of Urine and Other Symptomes wherewth Mr Potter is affected, I am perswaded that there is apprehended some Ulceration about the Neck of the Bladder wch perhaps may have penetrated into the Urethra so as to have corroded the Orifices of the Glandulae Prostates. The vomiting seems to proceed from a Consent of parts and is only Symptomatical therefore cannot think what Vomits or any other Remedies for cleansing ye Stomach be proper; such as are fitted to remove the Causes of the Vomiting wch from the pain in y^{r} side below ye Ribs I take to be a Gravel Stone adhering in the Ureter. If therefore the Vomiting and pain continue and you find his Pulse fall quick and strong, I think that it w^{d} be very proper to take 10 or 12 oz of Blood from his Arm either this Evening or tomorrow Morning as the Case may require, and afterward to administer the Anodyne Draught going to rest, if costive to make use of Glysters of Soothing decoctions, Herbs & Olive oil & Senna mixt with a Terebinth dissolved in ye Yolk of an Egg. Using Gaila Water with 3 scruples of Gum Arabic and Honey dissolved in each quart or Emulsions of ye cooling Laudanum 1 pt mixed with Gum Arabic: This Method to be pursued until the Vomiting and other Gravelly Symptoms cease. and then to begin again with the Pills and Tea already prescribed for his other Complaints. This Method I hope may have the desired Effect. As Circumstances may require I desire to hear further from you. I am wth best wishes for Mr Potter y^{r} Most Obed^{t}.

> Gum Arabic 3 scruples; Dissolve in 3 oz barley water and with 1 scruple of white poppy and 2 scruples senna. Make the Emulsion and add:
> Liquid Laudanum syrup 15 drops; Hollyhock syrup 3 scruples. Take part after bloodletting and repeat when doing it again.

Quer: Has Mr. Potter ever observed any Sudden Stoppage of Water.

[English]

Dr Sir,

I was favoured wth yours on friday Morning, but Mr. Potters vomiting had left him before & ye pain of his side not Violent, yet he finds it at times, but very little, his pulse was quite regular and loe so that I Omitted Bleeding him, as to that pricking pain in ye Anus he Complained off before has left him; but ye Sub-purulent Matter from ye Urethera continues as before, tho not in such quantitys. I gave him ye Draught at Bed time & rested very well, & ye Emulsion, and Barley Water with ye Gum sweetd with Honey for his Constant drink, yesterday in ye Eavening he Voided a Little Stone along with ye Sub-purulent Mater without any pains. Mr. Potter never finds any Sudden Stoppage of Urine & his Stomach is better, tomorrow Morning he proposes to take his Journey wch will be a Weak before he Return—and as soon as he return I shall give you an Acct—

in Haste yr Most Sincere Friend & Wellwisher to Command

John Simpson.

[Small sheet inserted.]

Mr. Dixon, aged 52.

Three years ago about February he was affected by a stroke at night and was left with dizziness, weakness and sluggishness, with a disposition to sleep. By autumn this lethargy greatly increased, and his sluggishness, with a great desire for rest.

March due to the lethargy, it had reached such a degree that he was rarely awake less than 8 hours in 24 and then with real drowsiness.

His complexion was white and he had an obese body, almost dropsical in nature; a feeble pulse. Appetite was good enough, thirst sometimes. His mouth often filled up with a sticky humour and his tongue was filthy—His Bowels worked normally. A white growth occupied his hand. His face was always cold and near a fire he shivered; loss of memory; weakness of sight.

[On the reverse of the sheet:]

Try to draw the viscid, thick, pituitous humours from the brain by using Setaces. Promote circulation of the blood and thin the humours by using Tinct. Veneris in Sal Volatile & diluted in an infusion of Water trefoil.

[Long, narrow piece of paper with an irregular edge. It is written in Latin with the writing very closed up.]

Epidemic Inflammatory Fever.[188]

Throughout the month of October 1737 from the end of September. The air suddenly grew cold with a storm followed by humid, wet air and little wind, then on the 16th October

[188] These observations on the epidemic fever sweeping Europe and Britain perhaps refer to typhus, a study that Brownrigg followed later in his medical career. They also indicate the close relationships which medical people assumed between weather and fever in the eighteenth century.

the air was clear and very cold, warm by day but freezing by night and this weather lasted without a break. The winds for all this time were northern winds from Europe or south winds from Europe.

During those days Mr. Creighton noted the Barometric reading of 17 was suddenly depressed, then rose above 18 on the 18th day only.

Over ⅓ of the inhabitants of Whitehaven fell ill with what was called Nervous Fever, Fever of the Spirit, Slow fever—it had raged before in Dublin, Newcastle, Bristol and other parts of Britain. Many of the people in Dublin were suddenly struck down and died without any warning and this was how this fever was brought to us, and before long similar fever was causing deaths in this place. Firstly, a shivering fit attacked, succeeded by heat with a rapid, fluttering pulse, a damp skin and profuse sweating, a moist tongue with the natural veinous colour sometimes white and black spots. Vomiting increased, lassitude and weakness crept over the whole body with intensive and often very vicious pains in the head and the back, and other general pains in the limbs with great chills. Coughs and difficulty in breathing. The blood showed signs of inflammation, sometimes with quinsy, pain, occasionally pleurisy but quite often eye problems. The feeling of cold was relieved by breath of fresh air, although the body still burned. Vomiting always after the application of solvent remedies. Dizziness grew twenty-fold as the fever increased. Frequent sneezing.

In children often in a coma, in weak bodies, infants emaciated by other illnesses, asthmatics, death is common. Nursing infants frequently perish. Apoplexy is the frequent mode of death for asthmatics. Old people and others are worn out before they die by the disease. The weather lasted without a break to the 7th November. On the 7th November the north wind blew from Europe and the skies were stirred with a warm wind and the air was humid and cloudy.

6. Warm air of 50° or more 7. Cold north wind. 8. Air now humid—temperature and winds varied. 12. Rain with the south winds.

[English]

An Account of the Weather at W^t^haven.

1736 Winter — Westerly Winds and strong Weather were every where common, so that the King was detained two months at Helvoit Sluyce by opposite winds, & bad weather[189] and the Virginia Ships could not sail from Whitehaven till the beginning of March. It was an exceedingly warm, open Winter, so that travelling from Harwich to London in January I saw Primroses, and rose trees shooting forth their leaves, & all the appearances of April.

[189] The relationship between the weather and illness was part of Brownrigg's thesis at Leiden. It was reported in the *Gentleman's Magazine* of 1737 that the King was indeed delayed in his return to England by adverse winds.

1736/7 Spring Inflammatory and intestinal fever, etc.	February was exceeding wet, we had cold frosty nights in April which nip the early Blossoms.
1737 Summer Various epidemic and nervous fevers with dysentery.	We had excessive hot Weather in the beginning of May wch might last about a fortnight, so that I observed the Thermometer often nigh eighty Digrees, the rest of the Summer was very dry, so that there was every where a great scarcity of Hey, but colder than usual with northerly Winds.
Autumn Common Dysentery.	The Months of Aug^{t} & 7^{ber} were pritty wet, altho the Weather continued pritty warm untill the latter end of September when it became suddenly very cold but about a week after it was a little warmer, and rainy and the Air very cloudy & thick and moist, and the mercury in Barometer was very low, on a sudden.
October 18th and Epidemic fever began to rage everywhere.	On Sunday the sixteenth of October the Air became clear serene and the Heat of the Sun a little warm in the daytime but in the Night was freezing cold. this kind of pleasant Weather lasted until the fourth of November, the Wind all this time being N.East. East and sometimes more Southerly. On the 7th of November the Wind N.
November Chest complaints and the same in February and January.	East the Sky cloudy, the Air became warm and very moist. On the 6th the Heat of the Air was 51 Digrees. On the 7th the Air was frosty, & clear with North Winds. On the 8th the Air was again moist with Southerly Winds, the Weather continued variable untill the middle of December when we had again three or four days of hard frost, to which suddenly succeeded a warm Thaw.
1737/8 February Scarlatina Spring 1738.	Spring generally cloudy & rainy with westerly Winds. Often thick Foggs especially in the beginning of May.
1738 Summer Erysipelas and similar fevers.	The Summer was excessive wet & rainy and moist and cold with westerly Winds, exceeding unseasonable Harvest Weather there scarce being a day thro the whole Summer entirely free from Rain, nor any Weather that was tolerably dry except about a fortnight towards the beginning of July.

Autumn Erysipelas Fevers.	The Autumn also was constantly wet & rainy with strong Westerly & Southerly Winds or thick foggy Weather. So that there were great floods, the low grounds being every where covered with Water. This kind of Weather continued till about the fifth of December.
Winter	About the fifth of Decemb: the Wind became Northerly the Air sharp & frosty, sometimes clear, sometimes foggy; but this weather did not last above ten or twelve days, after which we had almost perpetual Rains, with violent strong Winds, often doing great damage both by Sea and land, these Winds constantly blew from the South & South West Quarters. This sort of Weather held without Intermission till the beginning of March, we had therefore a warm open excessive wett & windy Winter.
1739 Spring	Mostly wet, sometimes warm and fair & pleasant especially in may.
Summer	Summer exceedingly wet & rainy & very cold with W and S.winds which continued from the latter end of May to September.
Autumn Nervous fevers quite slow, but rather infrequent. Weather otherwise very healthy, all through November.	About the beginning of September, the Easterly & Northerly winds began to blow & the weather became fair & clear but colder than usual at that Season, but good harvest weather in these parts; this continued till about the beginning of October when we had violent high Winds from the western quarter with thick haizy and rainy weather.
Winter Quite mild and diarrhoea very frequent.	About the middle of Octob: the eastern & Northern Winds began to blow and we had very little rain all the Winter after, there was a hard frost about the beginning of Novr and almost constantly at other times fine clear Weather.

APPENDIX I

LIST OF DOCTORS FROM EIGHTEENTH-CENTURY WHITEHAVEN

(Abstracted from P. J. Wallis and R. V. Wallis, *Eighteenth century medics: subscriptions, licences, apprenticeships*, Newcastle upon Tyne, Project for Historical Biobibliography, 1985.)

Date	*Name*	*Status*	*Apprentices*
1721–1790	AIREY, Thomas	M.D. (R)	–
1750 a1783	AIREY, Lancelot	M.D. (L)	–
b1675–1700	BARHAM, John	Apothecary	–
b1680 a1700	BECK, John	Apothecary	–
1745	BLENCOWE, Peter	Surgeon, etc.	BERM, Robert (S)
b1740 a1783	BRADLEY, John	Apothecary	–
1730 a1783	BRAGG, Joseph	Surgeon/Apothecary	–
1711–1780	BROWNRIGG, William	M.D. (L), F.R.S.E., F.R.S.	–
1765 b1829	CROSTHWAITE, Henry	M.D. (L)	–
–	CUNNINGHAM,	"Doctor"	–
b1780 a1829	DAWSON, Edward	Surgeon	–
1745–1825	DIXON, Joshua	M.D. (E), F.R.S.	–
1715 a1786	DIXON, Richard	M.D. (L)	–
1680–1729	DIXON, Thomas	M.D. (E)	–
b1780 a1799	ENGLAND, George	Druggist, Surgeon	
1722	GALE, Matthew	Surgeon	MORRIS, Charles (S)
b1655 a1696	GRAY, Francis	M.D.	–
b1755 a1822	GUNSON, Joseph	Army Surgeon	
1763	HAMBLETON, John	Surgeon	STEEL, Peter (S)
b1745 a1786	HAMILTON, John	Purveyor, Surgeon	MOORE, Thomas (S)
	HAMILTON, John	Purveyor, Surgeon	BORRADAILE, Jos (A)
	HAMILTON, John	Purveyor, Surgeon	RANKING, John (S/A)
1709–1780	HAMILTON, Isaac	Surgeon/Apothecary	DENTON, Edward (S)
	HAMILTON, Isaac	Surgeon/Apothecary	PUNCHON, George (S)
	HAMILTON, Isaac	Surgeon/Apothecary	MATHEWS, John (A)
	HAMILTON, Isaac	Surgeon/Apothecary	WYBERGH, William (S)
	HAMILTON, Isaac	Surgeon/Apothecary	BARWISE, John (A)
	HAMILTON, Isaac	Surgeon/Apothecary	DIXON, Richard (S)
	HAMILTON, Isaac	Surgeon/Apothecary	ROBINSON, Anthony (A)
	HAMILTON, Isaac	Surgeon/Apothecary	NICOLLSON, William (A)
	HAMILTON, Isaac	Surgeon/Apothecary	JOUART, Michael (S)
1678–1728	HESLOP, John	M.D. (L)	AIREY, Thomas (D/P)
1718	HISLOPP, John	D/P Apothecary	SENHOUSE, Patricius (A)
1743 a1786	JACKSON, John	Apothecary	–
1771–1817	JAMES, Hugh	M.D. (E)	–
	LITTLE	Surgeon	–
b1740 a1783	PEELE, John	Surgeon	STEELE, John (S)
	PEELE, John	Surgeon	HALL, Thomas (S)
	PEELE, John	Surgeon	SPEDDING, Demoivre (S)
1757	PEELE, Joseph	Apothecary	WILLIAMSON, John (A)
1735	SANDERSON, John	Surgeon	HINDLEY, George (S)
	SANDERSON, John	Surgeon	SHERMAN, Joseph (S)
1680 a1717	SENHOUSE, Richard	B.A., Apothecary	SMITH, Leopold (A)
	SENHOUSE, Richard	B.A., Apothecary	LATHES, William (A)
1722 a1748	SHAW, William	Apothecary	BULL, Edward (S)

1741	SMITH, Leonard	Apothecary	EDGCOMB, John (A)
1776–1865	STANLEY, John	M.D. (E)	–
1746–1785	STEEL, Henry	Medic	–
1755–1794	STEEL, John	Surgeon	–
1715	STEPHENSON, Thomas	Barber Surgeon	COOKE, John (B/S)
b1700 a1733	TOURVILLE, Charles	M.D.	–
b1750–1797	WILLIAMSON, Isaac	Surgeon/Apothecary	–
1780–1819	WILLIAMSON, Thomas	Naval Surgeon	–
1754	WYBERG, William	Apothecary	JACKSON, John (A)

b=before
a=after
(R) Graduated Rheims
(L) Graduated Leiden
(E) Graduated Edinburgh

(S) Surgeon
(A) Apothecary
(B/S) Barber Surgeon
(D/P) Doctor of Physick
(S/A) Surgeon Apothecary

Details of Whitehaven Practitioners

AIREY, Lancelot, M.D., Leiden. Thesis 'De Gonorrhoea Virulenta' 1st August 1772. Dedicated to his brother-in-law, the Rev. Wilford Huddleston of Whitehaven St. Nicholas. Author of *Symptoms, Nature and Causes and Cure of the Essera or Nettlerash* (Whitehaven, 1774).

AIREY, Thomas, M.D., Rheims. 1st February 1744. Father of Lancelot Airey. Died in Jamaica.

BROWNRIGG, William, M.D., Leiden. Thesis 'De Praxi Medica Ineunda' 18th January 1737. Dedicated to his Leiden teachers.

CROSTHWAITE, Henry, M.D., Leiden. Thesis 'De Rachitide' 22nd May 1789. Dedicated to Joseph Stamper, surgeon of Workington and William Allanby, M.D. Edinburgh.

DIXON, Richard, M.D., Leiden. Thesis 'De Phthisi Pulmonali' 11th December 1739.

HISLOP, John, M.D., Leiden. Thesis 'De Dentitione Infantum Difficili et Laboriosa'. Dedicated to his father Robert Heslopp, surgeon; Jabez Cary, M.D., chemist; and Oliver Horsman. M.D. 21st September, 1700.

SENHOUSE, Richard, M.D., unknown university, B.A. Oxford. Belonged to the Senhouse family of Netherhall, Maryport, Cumberland. Attended Leiden in 1717.

APPENDIX II

MEDICAL MEN MENTIONED IN THE CASEBOOK

Name	*Qualifications*	*Practice*
AMOS	"A Quack"	Whitehaven
ASKEW, Adam	M.D.	Newcastle
BARRY, Edward	F.R.S., F.C.P., M.D. (Leiden, Dublin, Oxford)	Cork
BENET, Timothy	M.D. (Leiden)	Norwich
BEWLEY, Thomas	Apothecary	Cockermouth
BOERHAAVE, Hermann	M.D. (Leiden), F.R.S.	Leiden
BOSWELL, John	M.D. (Leiden), F.R.S.E.	Edinburgh
BROWN, Henry	M.D. (Leiden)	Preston
BURTON, John	M.D. (Rheims), F.S.A.	York
CARLYLE, George	M.D. (Leiden)	Kendal
CHESELDEN, William	M.D., F.R.S. (Royal Surgeon)	Chelsea
CLEMENTSON, Wilfred	Surgeon/Apothecary	Cockermouth
COPE, Henry	M.D. (Dublin)	Dublin
COWPER, William	M.D. (Rheims), F.R.S.	London
CREIGHTON, Jonathan	Surgeon	Carlisle
FERN, James	Surgeon	London
FORLESSE	–	–
GARNIÈRE, Thomas	Apothecary	Chelsea College
GILCHRIST, Ebeneezer	M.D.	Dumfries
GREW, Nehemiah	M.D. (Leiden), F.R.S., F.C.P.	–
GRONOVIUS, Johannes	M.D. (Leiden)	Leiden
HALES, Stephen	D.D., F.R.S.	Teddington
HAMILTON, Isaac	Surgeon/Apothecary	Whitehaven
HARRISON, Peter	Surgeon/Apothecary	Preston
HARTLEY, David	M.D., F.S.A., F.R.S.	London
HAWKINS, George	M.R.C.S., F.S.A. (Royal Surgeon)	London
HAY, James	M.D. (Rheims)	Dumfries
HUTTON, John	M.D. (Padua), F.R.S., F.C.P., F.C.P.E.	Dumfries
KIRKPATRICK, James	M.D. (Glasgow)	Belfast
LAWSON, Isaac	M.D. (Leiden)	Flanders
LOBB, Theophilus	M.D. (Glasgow), F.R.S.	Shaftesbury
MEAD, Richard	M.D. (Padua), F.R.S., F.C.P.	London
MONRO, Alexander	M.D., F.R.S.E., F.R.S.	Edinburgh
MONROW, James	M.D., F.R.C.	London
PITTS, John	Surgeon	Devon
PLUMMER, Andrew	M.D. (Leiden), F.R.S.E., F.R.S., F.C.P.E.	Edinburgh
RADCLIFFE	–	–
SALKELD, Henry	M.D. (Rheims)	Whitehall
SANDERSON, John	Surgeon	London
SENHOUSE, Richard	Apothecary	Whitehaven
SHARP, Samuel	Surgeon	London
SHAW, Vessay	Surgeon	Dublin
SIMPSON, John	Apothecary	Cockermouth
SLARE, Frederick	M.D. (Utrecht), F.R.S., F.C.R.	Bath
SMELT, Thomas	M.B., M.D.	Stockton
SMITH, Leonard	Apothecary	Whitehaven

SWIETEN, Gerhard van	M.D. (Leiden)	Leiden
SYDENHAM, Thomas	M.B.	London
WALKER, Thomas	M.D. (Leiden)	York
WILLIS, Thomas	M.D., F.C.P., F.R.S.	Oxford
WOOD, John	–	–
WOODHOUSE, John	M.D. (Leiden)	Nottingham
WRIGHT, Robert	M.D. (Leiden)	–

APPENDIX III

LIST OF HERBS AND PLANTS USED BY BROWNRIGG

Casebook Reference	*Common Name*
Acacia	Gum Arabic
Acetos.	Sorrel
Actium Lappa	Burdock
Adiant.	Maidenhair
Aith.	Marshmallow
Aithamanta Oreoselinum	
Alium	Chive
Alkerm.	Kermes
Ammon.	Gum Ammoniac
Androm.	Erica
Aniseed	
Aristoloch.	Birthwort
Asparagus	
Attar	Oil of Roses
Aurant	Orange
Bal. Mar.	Costmary
Balsam	
Bardan.	Burberry
Beccabunga	Brooklime
Betonic	Water Betony
Calamit.	Calamint
Caryoph.	Clove–Pink
Cassia	Senna
Castan.	Chestnut
Cochiear	Horseradish
Consolid	Comfrey
Contrayerva	American Mulberry
Copaiva	Copaiba
Cucum.	Cucumber
Curcuma	Turmeric
Cydonia	Quince
Cynosb.	Rose Hip
Daucus	Wild carrot
Dealth.	Hollyhock
Diacod.	Poppy Heads
Diam.	Diamber
Enulcamp.	Elecampane
Eryng.	Sea Holly
Euphorb.	Spurge
Foen.	Fennel
Fragoselin.	Wild strawberry

Casebook Reference	*Common Name*
Fumaria	Fumitory
Funicae	Plantain Lily
Galingale	Umbrella plant Galingale
Genista	Broom
Glycyrrh.	Liquorice
Gram. Canin.	Twitchgrass
Guaiac.	Lignum Sanctum
Hedera	Ivy
Helenii	Elecampane
Helv.	Tincture of the styptic of Helvitius
Hord.	Barley
Hydrogalae	
Hypericum	St John's Wort
Hysop	Hyssop
Intybum	Chicory
Japon Terr.	Catechu
Lacca	Shellac
Lapath.	Sorrel
Lappa	Burdock
Lavand.	Lavender
Limon	Lemon
Lupula	Hop
Macid.	Mace
Maly.	Mallow
Man.	Flour
Mann.	Mandrake
Margarit	Pearl
Marubii	Horehound
Mastich.	Gum Mastic
Mecchocan	American Bindweed
Melilot	Yellow Melilot
Mille Folium	Yarrow
Nucia	Nut
Ocysum	Basil
Oliban.	Olibanum
Opopanac	Opopanax
Oryza	Rice

Paeon.	Paeony
Papav.	Poppy
Petrosilinum	Parsley
Plantag.	Plantain
Poterium	Salad Burnet
Prunus	Plum
Puleg.	Pennyroyal
Pyrethrum	Feverfew
Q.	Quince
Raphanus	Radish
Rhamni	Buckthorn
Rhei	Rhubarb
Rosar.	Rose
Rubia Tinctorum	Madder
Ruta	Rue
Sabinae	Savin
Sagapen.	Sagapenum
Sambuc.	Elderflower
Santal.	Sandalwood
Sem.	Houseleek
Serpent Virg.	Virginian snakeroot
Sinap.	Mustard
Styrac	Stryax
Taraxacum	Dandelion
Tinc. Croc.	Saffron
Tolutan	
Tussilago	Coltsfoot
Uvar.	Raisin
Uvar. Corinth.	Currant
Vaccin.	Hyacinth
Valerian Sylv.	Wild Valerian
Verbascum	Mullein
Veronica	
Vic.	Bean
Zingib.	Ginger

APPENDIX IV

WRITERS CITED BY BROWNRIGG

Petrus de Abano (1250–1316, *Epistulae*.
Aetius Amidenus (fl. *c*. 500), *De cognoscendis et curandis morbis*, Basle, 1533.
Michael Alberti (1682–1757), *Introductio in medicinam*, Halle, Orphanotropheum, 1721.
Amatus Lusitanus (1511–1568), *Curationum medicinalium centuriae septem*, Barcelona, S. and J. Mathevat, 1628.
Bartholomaeus Anglicus (d. 1260), *De proprietatibus rerum*, 1485.
Hieronymus Fabricius ab Aquapendente (1533–1619), *Operationes chirurgicae*, 1619.
Benedictus Aretius (1505–1574).
Aristotle (384–322 BC).
Hermann Boerhaave (1668–1738), *Aphorismi sive de cognoscendis et curandis morbis*, Leiden, J. van der Linden, 1715.
——*Atrocis nec descripti prius, morbi historia altera*, Leiden, S. Luchtmans, T. Haak, 1728.
——*Consultationes medicae*, London, J. Nourse, 1744.
Théophile Bonet (1620–1689), *Sepulchretum sive anatomia practica ex cadaveribus morbo denatis*, Geneva, Cramer and Perachon, 1700.
——*Medicina septentrionalis* (edition not identified).
Jacopus Bontius (1592–1631), *De medicina Indorum*, in P. Alpinus, *De medicina Aegyptiorum*, Paris, N. Redelichuysen, 1645.
Robert Boyle (1627–1691).
John Burton, *A treatise on the non-naturals*, York, A. Staples & J. Hildyard, 1738.
Barthélemy Cabrol (b. 1529), *Alphabet Anatomie*, Tournon, C. Michel and G. Linocier, 1594.
C. Dellon (b. *c*. 1649), *Nouvelle relation d'un voyage fait aux Indes orientales*, Amsterdam, F. Marret, 1699.
Marcellus Donatus (1538–d. *c*. 1600), *De historia medica*, Frankfurt, J. J. Porsius, 1613.
Bartholomaeus Eustachius (1520–1574), *Opuscula anatomica*, Venice, V. Luchinus, 1564.
Petrus Forestus (1522–1597), *Observationes et curationes medicinales*, Leiden, F. Raphelengius, 1596.
J. Freind (1675–1728), *Opera omnia*, London, J. Wright, 1733.
Galen (129–*c*.200 AD).
Stephen Hales (1677–1761).
David Hartley (1705–1757), *A view of the present evidence for and against Mrs. Stephens's Medicines*, London, S. Harding, 1739.
Walter Harris (1647–1732), *De morbis acutis infantum*, Amsterdam, J. F. Bernard, 1715.
Johann Hartmann (1568–1631), *Praxis chimiatrica*, 1633.
William Harvey (1578–1659), *De motu cordis et sanguinis*, 1628.
Hippocrates (*c*. 460–377 BC), ed. A. Foesius, *Opera*, Frankfurt, Heirs of A. Wechel, 1595. [References in notes to *Oeuvres complètes d'Hippocrate*, ed. É. Littré, 10 vols, Amsterdam, Adolf M. Hakkert, 1973–89.]
Jacobus Hollerius (d. 1562), *Opera omnia practica*, Paris, J. Dallin, 1664.
Gregor Horst (1578–1636), *Opera medica*, 3 vols, Gouda, G. van der Hoeve, 1661.
Ulrich von Hutten (1488–1523).
Titus Lucretius Carus (*c*. 98–55 BC).
Theophilus Lobb, *On dissolvents of the stone . . .*, London, J. Buckland, 1739.
Marcello Malpighi (1628–1694).
Pietro de Marchettis (1589–1673).
Valentin Andreas Moellenbrock (d. 1675), *De varis seu arthritide vage scorbutica tractatus*, Leipzig, G. Michaelis for J. Gross, 1672.
Moschion (after 500 AD), *De passionibus mulierum liber graecus*.

Johannes Ott of Schaffhausen (1639–1717).
Ambroise Paré (1510–1590).
Severinus Pinaeus (d. 1619), *De integritatis et corruptionis virginum notis.*
Nicolaus Piso (d. 1590), *De cognoscendis et curandis praecipue internis humani corporis morbis*, Leiden, Q. Visser, 1736.
Felix Plater (1538–1614), *Observationes, in hominis affectibus*, Basil, L. König, 1641.
John Radcliffe (1652–1714).
John Ray (1627–1705).
Lazare Rivière (1589–1655), *Observationes medicae et curationes insignes*, in *Opera medica universa*, either Lyons, J. Hugueton, 1679, or, Lyons, Anisson and J. Posuel, 1698.
Gulielmus Rondeletius (1507–1566).
Balduinus Ronsseus (1525–1597), *De magnis Hippocratis lienibus... seu... scorbuto commentarius*, in D. Sennertus, *De scorbuto*, Frankfort & Wittenberg, Heirs of T. Marius, & E. Schumacher, 1654.
Frederik Ruysch (1638–1731).
Giovanni Domenico Santorini (1681–1737), *Opuscula medica de structu & motu fibrae*, Rotterdam, 1719.
Laurentius Scholz (1681–1737), *Epistulae philosophicae*, Hanover, Wechel, 1610.
Melchior Sebizius (1664–1704), *Manualis sive speculum medicinae*, Strassburg, F. Spoor, 1661.
Daniel Sennert (1572–1637), *Practicae medicinae liber primus (—sextus)*, Paris, 1633.
——*De scorbuto*, Frankfort & Wittenberg, Heirs of T. Marius, & E. Schumacher, 1654.
Reinert Solenander (1524–1601), *Consilia medicinalia*, Frankfurt, Heirs of Wechel, C. Marnius, & J. Aubrius, 1596.
Paul de Sorbait (1624?–1691), *Universa medicina*, Nuremberg, J. and F. Endter, 1672.
Georg Ernst Stahl (1660–1734), *De motu haemorrhoidali, et fluxu haemorrhoidum*, Paris, 1730.
——*Theoria medica vera*, Halle, 1708, 2nd ed. 1721.
——*Abhandlung von der goldenen Ader*, Leipzig, 1729.
Thomas Sydenham (1624–1689), *Opera universa*, Leiden, J. Kerchem, 1726.
Franciscus Deleboe Sylvius (1614–1672), *Praxis medica.*
Philip Verheyen (1648–1710), *Corporis humani anatomia libri humani*, Brussels, Serstevens, 1726.
Bernhard Verzascha (1628–1680), *Observationum medicarum centuria*, Basle, J. J. Decker for H. Wetstenius, 1677.
Andreas Vesalius (1514–1564), *De humani corporis fabrica*, Basle, J. Oporinus, 1543.
Johannes Walaeus (1604–1649), *Epistulae duae de motu chyli et sanguinis.*
Thomas Willis (1621–1675), *Pharmaceutice rationalis*, The Hague, A. Leer, 1677.
J. Woodhouse, *Dissertatio de medicina instituenda et promovenda*, Leiden, 1700.

APPENDIX V

List of books in Sir James Lowther's Library, Flatt Hall
13.10.1757–by Thomas Ashburner

FOLIO	MEDICAL BOOKS	
228	Wiseman's Surgery	London 1676
235	Riverius's Practice of Physick, etc.	London 1661
236	Riverius's Practice of Physick, etc.	London 1685
237	Democritus's Anatomy of Melancholy	London 1660
238	Shape's Anatomy	London 1683
239	Charras's Royal Pharmocopeia	London 1687
244	Bonet's Guide to the Practical Physician	London 1684
248	Parey's Surgery	London 1634
249	Pharmacopeia Londinensis	London 1650
250	Riolanus's Anatomy	London 1671
251	Senertus on the Venereal Pox, etc.	London 1660
323	Gerrard's Herbal	1636
330	Bidloo's Anatomy	Amsterdam 1685
QUARTO		
35	The School of Salerno	London 1634
69	Veslignii Syntagma anatomicum	Batavii 1647
140	Edward's Chirugery Plain	London 1636
223	Barrhough's Method of Physick	London 1652
332	Lister's Exercitatio Anatomica, etc.	London 1696
277	Sydenham on The Gout. A Manuscript (Leather Bound)	
OCTAVO		
13	Lister Exercitationes Medicales	London 1697
23	Anatomy Epitomised	London 1682
25	Dr. Willis's Practice of Physick	London 1685
133	Natural History of Poisons	Savoy 1674
152	Roonhuyse's Treatise on the Gout	London 1676
187	Sperrie's House of Medicines	London 1686
202	The Compleat Chymist	London 1677
224	Lovel's Herbal	Oxford 1665
271	Sydenham Tractus de Podagra, etc.	London 1683
356	L'Instinct de Medicine	
422	Heurnii Institutiones Medicinae	
509	Lister Exercitatio Anatomica	
578	Sebertus's Whole Art of Physick & Surgery	
623	The Conckave of Physicians	
654	Levini Lemnii Medici Terezei de Habitu	
730	Sherley's Treatise of the Gout	
731	Rowzee's Treatis of Tunbridge Waters	
733	Taylor's Wonderfull Secret in Curing Agues and Fevers	
740	Read's Anatomy	
753	Peter's Treatise of Dulwich Wells	
778	Helvetii Physicarum	
781	Hippocrates Aphorisms	
850	Spink's Sick Man Visited	

911	Glissonii Anatomia Hepatis
915	Antonides de Scriptis Medicis
924	Colebatch on the Gout
925	A collection of Acute Diseases
999	Thurguet on the Gout
1021	Streater on the Veneral Pox and Gout
1166	Roonhuyse on the Gout
1167	A treatise on the Gout and Kings Evil
1183	Rules of Health
1206	The Doctor and Student Abridged (1687)
1214	Rules of Health
1264	Hieronimi Medici de Subtilitate
1299	The Cure of the Smallpox
1302	Bartholini Anatomica
1303	Jones on Opium

INDEX